Praise for *The Estrogen Fix*

"*The Estrogen Fix* offers an easy-to-read explanation that removes the confusion regarding how to safely take estrogen. Once women realize they have an estrogen window, they can take back control of their lives."

—**Sara Gottfried, MD,** author of *New York Times* bestselling books *The Hormone Reset Diet* and *The Hormone Cure*

"Dr. Seibel's meticulous review of the most recent scientific evidence about menopausal hormones will help the reader think about the extra benefits that result from taking estrogen in the right way and at the right time. Clearly presented, this book shows that estrogen therapy improves quality of life including workability, prevents disease, and can be life-saving."

—**Philip M. Sarrel, MD,** professor emeritus of obstetrics, gynecology, and reproductive sciences and professor emeritus of psychiatry, Yale University School of Medicine

"I couldn't put this book down! I have been longing for a doctor to write a book that will help women clearly understand the benefits of estrogen, when to use it, and how. Most women are still basing their health care on fear instead of facts. Dr. Seibel walks us through the impact of estrogen on our breasts, heart, brain, bones, vagina, bladder, and skin! Thank you, Dr. Seibel, for giving us all the information, studies, and tools to help keep us healthy and happy through menopause and beyond."

—**Ellen Dolgen,** speaker, author, blogger, and health and wellness advocate; founder and president of Menopause Mondays at EllenDolgen.com

"In his new book, *The Estrogen Fix*, Mache Seibel, MD, has created a breakthrough guide to coach women through menopause. He clarifies how to manage menopause symptoms, balance the risks and benefits of hormone therapy and when might be the best time to consider treatment, and how to communicate effectively with your doctor. Highly recommended for anyone dealing with menopause issues."

—**Steven Masley, MD, FAHA, FACN, FAAFP, CNS,** bestselling author of *Smart Fat* and *The 30-Day Heart Tune-Up* and creator of top public television programs: *30 Days to a Younger Heart* and *Smart Fats to Outsmart Aging.*

"In *The Estrogen Fix,* Dr. Mache Seibel tells us everything
we need to know about one of the most frequently prescribed
medications in America. The crucial message is one women
have known for millennia: Timing is everything."

–**Julie Holland, MD,** author of *Moody Bitches: The Truth About the Drugs You're Taking,
the Sleep You're Missing, the Sex You're Not Having, and What's Really Making You Crazy*

"*The Estrogen Fix* is a book very much needed among women today,
many of whom suffer not only from the effects of their menopause,
but even more from the effects of misinformation.
Dr. Seibel has written a clear, concise, readable, and knowledgeable
source of information. One that will be immediately valuable to the
many women and their families who suffer from estrogen deprivation."

–**Ricardo Azziz, MD, MPH;** Regents' professor, Georgia Regents
University; former founding president, Georgia Regents University; former
president, Georgia Health Sciences University; former founding
CEO, Georgia Regents Health System

"Dr. Mache Seibel has made a major contribution to women's health
in writing *The Estrogen Fix.* As both a scientific expert on menopause
and an expert in communicating to women, he has beautifully
clarified the confusing topic of should women take estrogen as they go
through menopause. Dr. Mache offers the data and puts it into a
perspective that will explain safe usage of the most effective therapy for
menopausal symptoms. All women making choices
on menopausal interventions will benefit from reading this book."

–**Mary Jane Minkin, MD, FACOG, NCMP;** clinical professor of obstetrics,
gynecology and reproductive sciences, Yale School of Medicine

The Estrogen Fix

The Breakthrough Guide to Being Healthy, Energized, and Hormonally Balanced—Through Perimenopause, Menopause, and Beyond

MACHE SEIBEL, MD

Creator of the Menopause Quiz (www.MenopauseQuiz.com)
and founder of *The Hot Years* magazine (www.HotYearsMag.com)

RODALE.

RODALE *wellness*

Live happy. Be healthy. Get inspired.

Sign up today to get exclusive access to our authors, exclusive bonuses, and the most authoritative, useful, and cutting-edge information on health, wellness, fitness, and living your life to the fullest.

Visit us online at RodaleWellness.com
Join us at RodaleWellness.com/Join

Rodale books may be purchased for business or promotional use or for special sales. For information, please email BookMarketing@Rodale.com.

Printed in the United States of America
Rodale Inc. makes every effort to use acid-free ♾, recycled paper ♻.

Illustrations by Paige Vickers

Book design by Carol Angstadt

Library of Congress Cataloging-in-Publication Data is on file with the publisher.
ISBN 978–1–63565–012–9 trade paperback

Distributed to the trade by Macmillan
2   4   6   8   10   9   7   5   3   1

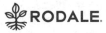

Follow us @RodaleBooks on 🐦 f 𝓟 ⊚

We inspire health, healing, happiness, and love in the world.
Starting with you.

To my wife, Sharon, for providing me with the "why" for writing it and for all her unconditional love, help, and support while seeing it through.

Also to women everywhere who are struggling with the question of whether or not to take estrogen. Once you understand your estrogen window, you will be able to talk confidently with your health-care provider, decide whether estrogen is right for you, and receive your estrogen fix.

Contents

Introduction

If you are confused about and afraid to take estrogen, if you're taking estrogen and hoping you haven't made a dangerous mistake, if you're not taking estrogen and want to discover what its impact could be on your health, or if you are comfortable with your decision to take estrogen and just want to know more about it, *The Estrogen Fix* is the book for you. It will eliminate your confusion, calm your fears, and answer all your questions. And answers to questions about estrogen are desperately needed.

All you have to do is mention "estrogen" or "hormone therapy" (HT) to women and you'll get a wide range of reactions, from "Estrogen saved my life during menopause" to "I hear hormone therapy can cause breast cancer." Since prescription estrogen was first introduced in 1942 to treat the symptoms of menopause, it has been called everything from a fountain of youth and a preventive for osteoporosis and heart disease to a cause of uterine cancer and dementia. At various times, estrogen has been vilified as a cause of breast cancer or heralded as a guard against breast cancer. No wonder women and their doctors are so confused.

These inconsistent and contradictory reports have left women believing that using estrogen is a medical form of Russian roulette, a treatment that could likely relieve their symptoms but could potentially cost them their health or even their lives. Unfortunately, that kind of misinformation has caused millions of women to avoid estrogen or to take it with trepidation—"Hormone therapy may save my life, but I've read so many articles and blog posts about how the stuff is toxic that I'm scared and would rather suffer with my menopause symptoms than take it."

Nothing could be further from the truth. Hormone therapy is safe and beneficial for the majority of women. I want you to know that and why.

Whether or not you decide to take estrogen is the most important midlife medical decision you, as a woman, will make. Why do I say that? Because whether or not you take estrogen will affect almost every part of your body—your skin, weight, breasts, brain, bones, bladder, mood, vagina, libido, and a whole lot more. Your decision will change your risk of major health conditions like osteoporosis, breast cancer, and dementia. Your choice will affect the quality of your sex life, mood, memory, skin, and weight control as well as the quality of your work. I want you to be so well informed that you can decide whether or not to take estrogen with confidence and clarity. Helping women understand the power of estrogen is my passion. It's why I wrote *The Estrogen Fix*.

Why am I so passionate about this topic? It started well over a decade ago when my wife, Sharon, found out she had the BRCA or BReast CAncer gene that increased her risk of breast and ovarian cancers. She had both her ovaries and her fallopian tubes removed in February 2003 at an early age and immediately went into menopause. Because she was at increased risk of breast cancer, her doctors felt she would only be able to take estrogen for 5 years at most. But my own research suggested she could and should take estrogen for a longer period of time, and her forward-thinking gynecologist agreed too. That's when I began trying to understand the estrogen window and the estrogen fix; I needed to figure out whether Sharon could be on estrogen for an extended period of time, because I believed the benefits greatly outweighed the risks. The general consensus at that time was that Sharon should not continue taking estrogen for the long term because of the results of the 2002 Women's Health Initiative study, which I talk about below and which had been published only 7 months earlier.

I remember July 9, 2002, like it was yesterday. I was seeing patients in my office just outside Boston, and the phones started ringing off the hook. My receptionists couldn't keep up as patient after patient called in a panic to find out what I thought of that day's headline, "Hormone Replacement Study a Shock to the Medical System." It was the report heard round the world.

This enormous reaction was in response to the terrifying news from the first Women's Health Initiative study, or WHI, published in the *Journal of the American Medical Association*. The first WHI study was on the risks and benefits of taking a combo pill called Prempro that contained the estrogen Premarin plus the synthetic progesterone Provera (medroxyprogesterone acetate–MPA). That combo treatment was called estrogen-progestogen therapy or EPT. The WHI was prematurely discontinued because Prempro reportedly caused an increased risk of breast cancer, heart attacks, blood clots, and stroke. Every woman who was taking any form of estrogen at that time was concerned. And we're talking about millions and millions of women. It was a very long day that overflowed into the weeks and months to come.

I'm not sure how many of my patients threw away their estrogen that day, or how many millions of women around the globe stopped taking Prempro, but I do know that day in 2002 marked the beginning of a medical tsunami. Women and their doctors were caught in a crossfire of anger, fear, distrust, suffering, and a lack of answers. Estrogen was and is the most effective treatment for most of the symptoms of menopause. But after the 2002 WHI report was published, every patient visit included a question something like, "Should I be taking estrogen or not? If I take it, will I get breast cancer and die?"

In 2004 a second WHI report was published that evaluated the risks and benefits of the estrogen Premarin without Provera, called estrogen therapy or ET, and the results were strikingly different. Estrogen alone was given to women who had had a hysterectomy. They did not need Provera to prevent estrogen from causing cancer of the uterine lining. I'll explain more about this later. What's important to understand is that the 2004 WHI study found that Premarin taken alone did not cause an increased risk of breast cancer and might actually decrease breast cancer risk. Premarin alone also didn't increase the risk of heart disease.

Unfortunately, the media and many health-care providers did not distinguish between the risks and benefits of Premarin versus Prempro or the age at which either of these medications was begun. So women were led to believe that using estrogen in any form was a losing proposition. Even if the treatment could likely relieve their menopausal symptoms, it could potentially cost them their health or even their lives. More and more women began thinking, "My symptoms are making me uncomfortable, embarrassed, miserable, tired, foggy, less interested in sex, less effective at work, gain weight, or incredibly moody (you fill in the blank), but they won't last forever. I can tough it out."

How do *you* feel about estrogen? Are you certain that whatever the benefits, no matter how great, it isn't worth the risk and worry of taking it? Perhaps you are like my patient Jennifer, who came in saying, "I'm not taking estrogen. I'm a strong woman; I can get through this."

I want to change that mind-set. The existing way of thinking has created a brain drain for women—nearly 15 years of menopausal side effects that could have been avoided and that, as you will discover, have robbed millions of women of quality of life and advancement at work. That is why it's so important for you to be informed.

Or are you afraid or confused to consider taking estrogen because of the things you've heard about it? Are you wondering, "Is estrogen safe for me? Is it worth the potential risks? How long should I take it? Which one? What dose? When should I start taking it? When should I stop taking it? Why doesn't somebody figure this out and explain it to me so I won't have to worry?" *The Estrogen Fix* answers all these questions and more, so you'll be empowered with the right facts and knowledge to discuss with your doctor or other health-care provider. Given the current level of confusion, the more you understand, the more likely you will be to get the right treatment, or for that matter, any treatment at all.

As a physician who specializes in this area, I've watched as a generation of women and their health-care providers struggled with those same questions and concerns. It's no wonder. Many newer medical reports have come out since the first WHI study that also suggested taking estrogen is a huge risk. And once something becomes a "fact," opinions change slowly. But before the 2002 WHI report, the truth then was that estrogen was safe and helpful for almost all women. And then suddenly it wasn't.

As Mark Twain once said, "All generalizations are inaccurate, including this one." I was determined to figure out why there was so much confusion about estrogen. I needed to know for Sharon and for my patients. How could the same medication that was so helpful and lowered the risk of certain diseases also be dangerous and a ticking medical time bomb? After looking more carefully at the original 2002 WHI report and culling nuggets of information from it and the 2004 study and from hundreds of other reports, as well as continuously interviewing the authors who wrote most of those papers in my capacity as editor of *The Hot Years* magazine, I uncovered piece after piece of a large puzzle. I found a different truth—one that made sense out of all the confusion.

There are two parts to understanding the estrogen window. The first is that Prempro and Premarin are two very different medications, and as you will learn, they present two very different sets of risks. It was the Provera in the Prempro not Premarin that was associated with most of the negative findings, which I explain later. The second part is to eliminate the remaining confusion, contradiction, and consternation—a simple concept that explains how to minimize the risks and negative findings about estrogen yet maximize its benefits. It is a concept so simple to understand that by the end of *The Estrogen Fix* you will be empowered with the knowledge to decide whether estrogen is a treatment that you could and should consider with confidence. In fact, you'll discover that NOT taking estrogen may *increase* your risk of the very illnesses that are currently making you avoid it.

After reading *The Estrogen Fix* you won't have to feel that treating your most worrisome menopausal symptoms that are lowering the quality and quantity of your life randomly exposes you to serious risks. All you have to do is understand that you have an estrogen window—a window of time in which estrogen poses minimal risks and maximum benefits; after that window of time closes, outcomes change, and estrogen can expose you to lesser benefits with potentially much greater risks. It's the secret you'll uncover to achieve your estrogen fix.

With what you discover in *The Estrogen Fix* you will be able to understand how the information about taking estrogen became so confusing, why it doesn't have to be that way, and how estrogen can improve your life. You'll understand the differences between Premarin (or other estrogens taken alone) and Prempro (or combinations of estrogen plus natural or synthetic progesterone) and the differences between oral and transdermal (through the skin) and synthetic and bioidentical estrogen. You'll also understand when estrogen is *not* the best choice for you and discover alternative treatments that may help you reduce your symptoms. And that is really good news, because once you discover your estrogen window, you won't feel you have to "grin and bear" the hot flashes, brain fog, vaginal dryness, weight gain, and other symptoms of menopause. You won't have to unknowingly expose your body to an increased risk of Alzheimer's disease, heart disease, osteoporosis, breast cancer, and early aging of skin. Whether you are in perimenopause, early menopause, menopause, or postmenopause, you will know how to discuss ET and EPT with your health-care provider. You will become a messenger for helping your friends and family members get the treatment they need.

It's time to stop "treatment as usual." It's time to stop depending on whether your health-care provider has time or the latest information to help you determine if estrogen is right for you. With the information you are about to discover, you will be able to evaluate estrogen as you would any treatment option and have a good idea whether it is a good choice or too risky. You'll be able to choose ET or EPT logically. Consider this graphic:

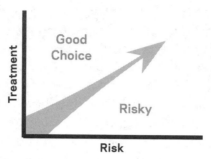

You should be able to consider your treatment and decide whether it is a good choice or a risky one for you. Imagine how empowering that will feel.

For well more than a decade, millions of women have avoided taking any form of estrogen, and a surprising percentage of health-care providers still avoid prescribing it. As you read through *The Estrogen Fix*, you will discover that not taking estrogen in some instances can have some significant negative effects on your health that you can avoid. With this book, your estrogen window will be thrown wide open, so a new conversation about the benefits of Premarin or Prempro (or their comparables) can begin. Some doctors are once again beginning to endorse estrogen for appropriate candidates with significant symptoms. We are entering another major transition era in women's health, and when armed with the information in *The Estrogen Fix* you will be at the forefront of the discussion and can help lead the way.

The point of *The Estrogen Fix* is not to tell all women to take estrogen or that estrogen is right for you. But once you have the knowledge and awareness raised in *The Estrogen Fix*, you can talk to your health-care provider. My goal is to raise awareness of the estrogen window so that if you want to take estrogen to help alleviate your symptoms or to prevent certain diseases, you will understand that there is a window of opportunity—the estrogen window—in which taking estrogen can be highly effective with the least potential for a negative outcome. Imagine really understanding the issues surrounding estrogen so that you are not afraid or anxious about taking it. Imagine feeling in control and comfortable about your decision.

Estrogen and estrogen plus progesterone or synthetic progesterone will be explained in detail, but for now, know that estrogen is a naturally occurring hormone that affects almost every organ in a woman's body. I'm going to go through each issue (brain, breasts, heart, bones, weight, skin, bladder, vagina) and tell exactly how estrogen will positively affect each one.

As astrophysicist Neil deGrasse Tyson said when discussing America's first trip to the moon, "We went to the moon and we discovered the earth." With *The Estrogen Fix*, I want you to learn about your estrogen window and through that, discover how estrogen can affect your entire body and your future health. You will learn the good about estrogen, the bad about it, and most importantly, the timing of it. And that will empower you to achieve your estrogen fix.

How important is estrogen? Estrogen stimulates growth and renewal in tissues as diverse as bone, brain, bladder, skin, and vagina. If taken at the right time, estrogen improves bloodflow, brings nutrition and oxygen to cells, removes free radicals, and fights inflammation. Think of estrogen as playing a supporting role in maintaining the female body's ecosystem. Lower estrogen levels are responsible for the hot flashes, night sweats, weight gain, and vaginal dryness of menopause that affect so many women. But even more insidiously, low levels of estrogen can take a toll on most of the body's organs. When production begins to decrease or stops completely as women head into, through, and beyond menopause, the tissues that estrogen once supported slowly break down. Falling estrogen levels also increase a woman's risk of heart disease, Alzheimer's disease, and other cognitive issues, and osteoporosis and resulting bone fractures. These dangerous conditions come with the risk of two unpleasant side effects: lower quality of life and premature death.

Yet as a longtime Harvard-educated ob-gyn who has spent nearly 20 years teaching at Harvard and nearly another decade at the University of Massachusetts directing the Complicated Menopause Program, and who has treated more than 10,000 patients, I've found that when it comes to menopause, there exists a pervasive fear of dying prematurely as a result of *taking* supplemental estrogen. This thinking often leads women to refuse ET and EPT that contain estrogen, and for many of their doctors to refuse to prescribe it. For the sake of clarity and accuracy, we're going to talk about estrogen only and estrogen plus either progesterone or synthetic progesterone as two different things.

The research I've done has allowed me to help Sharon and thousands of my patients. Now I want to help you and share with you a new way to think about estrogen and how to approach whether or not estrogen is right for you. By conducting a broad review and analysis, I was able to create a complete and accurate picture about estrogen and menopause. The results: There are two different types of estrogen-containing medications, and there is a safe way to use them that maximizes their benefits and minimizes their risks. And when to take estrogen and gain its benefits has to do with knowing when your individual estrogen window is open. Imagine that instead of worrying about whether or not to take estrogen as though the risks and benefits were gambling at a casino, you could know your best individual window to most safely gain the potential benefits before that window closes. And if you take advantage of your estrogen window, you will increase your chances of improving the quality of your physical and mental health, and you won't have to endure all the ongoing unpleasant symptoms of menopause.

Most of the two million American women who enter menopause each year want to know how to alleviate their disruptive menopausal symptoms. When estrogen is the answer, women are reluctant to take it, because they have heard so many negative things about it. Likewise, many health-care providers avoid mentioning estrogen because they are relying on outdated information about perceived risks. Perhaps they don't have time for a lengthy discussion on estrogen therapy. Or, given how busy they are and their limited amount of time, they are doing the best they can, but they don't know when their patients should take estrogen to gain lifelong benefits.

The Estrogen Fix explains that women who replace lost estrogen at a specific time in their lives, during their estrogen window, can minimize the debilitating symptoms of menopause and enjoy a healthy, vibrant life. *The Estrogen Fix* also answers the question, "*When* should I take estrogen to gain the most benefits?" Taking ET or EPT as the body's natural production begins to decrease has repeatedly been shown to be the most protective and effective opportunity.

The Estrogen Fix:

- Shows you how to determine the best time for you to take estrogen-containing medications and which are the best treatment options for you

- Explains why millions of women unnecessarily and prematurely abandoned Premarin and Provera that were protecting them from breast cancer, heart disease, dementia, and more

- Clarifies the risks and benefits of estrogen and how to know whether estrogen is right for you

- Answers your questions and prepares you to speak with your doctor about ET and EPT and heart disease, osteoporosis, dementia, and more

- Anchors a personal menopause breakthrough with understanding your estrogen window so you don't have to "grin and bear" the symptoms and consequences of menopause

Throughout *The Estrogen Fix*, I refer to the symptoms and stories of specific patients. To protect their identities, I've changed their names and combined their stories into composites of the thousands of patients I've treated. But all the patient comments and examples are ones I've heard over and over and are used to illustrate a point, and they will help you identify examples of the very things you may be coping with in your life.

When you look at recently published books on the topic of menopause, just a few mention estrogen in the title, even though falling estrogen levels produce the symptoms—hot flashes, night sweats, mood swings, irritability, brain fog, fractured sleep, and sexual issues—that plague women during this time. With the most recent research and newest information, *The Estrogen Fix* takes the emotions out of your decision and sets the record straight about how ET and EPT can have positive effects if *taken at the right time* of this new stage of life.

The Estrogen Fix shows you the many positive things that estrogen can do for your body and total well-being before, during, and after menopause. When the details of the WHI study were released in 2002, I watched as hundreds of my patients threw away their estrogen-containing medications. And they suffered. If they had known what you are about to read in *The Estrogen Fix*, their lives would have been happier and healthier. That's what I want for you. And the sooner you educate yourself, the more opportunities you have to protect your health and the health of your friends and family, and prevent the very diseases that a lack of estrogen can cause. And that will be transformative.

Chapter 1

Estrogen: Behind the Headlines

In the 35 years that I've been a doctor and women's health specialist, estrogen has gone from hero to zero and back and forth again. How could this happen? How could the most frequently prescribed medication in America fall out of favor overnight? How could the same medication be so good and so bad, so loved and so hated, so beneficial and so harmful?

In this chapter we go behind the headlines and pull back the curtain to see how we got to this point and the circuitous path that took us there. Once the information becomes clear, it will be easy to understand how estrogen was blamed for problems it wasn't responsible for. The main characters in this story are Premarin (an estrogen only), which we'll call the "good guy," and Prempro (Premarin plus Provera), which we'll call the "bad guy." Prempro is a medication distinctly different from Premarin, though it contains Premarin, and as a result, Prempro has risks and benefits different from those of Premarin alone. I'll explain what these are later in the book and how to deal with them. I'll also show you how the estrogen window influences both of them.

The story begins at the end of a woman's reproductive years, when her reproductive hormones estrogen and progesterone transition from well-synchronized to unbalanced cycles that become progressively more unpredictable as she ages. During that window of time, estrogen levels fall, and the symptoms so typical of menopause begin to appear—hot flashes, vaginal dryness, embarrassing bladder symptoms, lower libido,

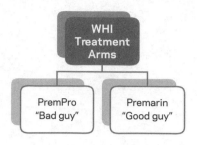

poor sleep, and more. It just makes sense that since all this happens as estrogen levels are falling, giving estrogen at that time would help decrease those symptoms—and it does.

So for several decades, doctors prescribed estrogen to women to relieve their perimenopausal and menopausal symptoms. But the plot thickens, because as I mentioned previously, there are two main characters, two hormones: estrogen and progesterone. I'll explain this in detail in the section on the history of estrogen.

If you look at a graph of the estrogen and progesterone levels during perimenopause, which is the time leading up to and just beyond menopause, it would look like a graph of the Dow Jones heading from a bull market into a recession. The zigzagging ups and downs trend downward and eventually remain low for the rest of a woman's life.

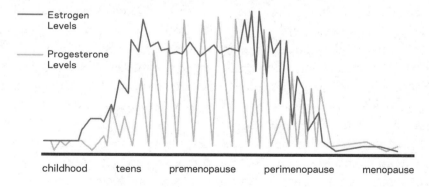

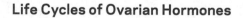

Perimenopause and early menopause are the times when most women start taking estrogen-containing medications, such as Premarin and Prempro. Women traditionally *began* taking these medications within the first 10 years of entering menopause, because that's when their symptoms are usually worst.

So why did the Women's Health Initiative (WHI) studies decide to give some women Premarin and others Prempro, and why did most of the women begin receiving medication between the ages of 60 and 79? It all depended on whether or not each woman still had her uterus. As you will see, this is a key point for understanding your estrogen window and how all the confusion got started.

Estrogen taken alone can lead to changes in the cells of the uterine lining over time; over a decade or more, these can turn into endometrial cancer. So Premarin, which is estrogen only, could not be safely used in women who had not had a hysterectomy. The good news is that if progesterone or a substance that acts in the body like progesterone (called a progestogen) is added, the risk of cancer of the uterine lining is virtually eliminated. So when the WHI studies were designed, women who had not had a hysterectomy were given Prempro, which contained Premarin and Provera. Women who had their uterus removed by hysterectomy were given Premarin (estrogen only).

Progesterone is the name of a hormone your body makes. Its name comes from "pro-gestation," because it prepares the uterine lining, which has been primed with estrogen, to receive and support a pregnancy. The use of Provera rather than progesterone in combination with estrogen in the WHI studies is what caused most of the problems and confusion about the risks and benefits of estrogen. As mentioned on page 1, Provera is the "bad guy."

At the beginning of the WHI studies, progesterone was not available as a pill, but Provera was, so that was prescribed. Prempro, which contained Premarin plus Provera, was a very popular pill at the time. Provera, like progesterone, is a *progestogen*, the term applied to any hormone that acts like progesterone in the body. Provera is the brand name for medroxyprogesterone acetate or MPA, a synthetic progestogen. Synthetic progestogens are called progestins. This incredibly confusing nomenclature is made even worse because when writing articles, many people use these terms interchangeably and incorrectly. A short biochemistry discussion will make a lot of things clearer when we discuss the WHI in more detail. The flow diagram on page 4 will help clarify the information. While there are other synthetic progestins, I'll limit the discussion to Provera for now.

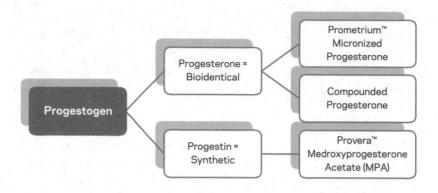

The Women's Health Initiative

In 1991, the WHI under the aegis of the US National Institutes of Health (NIH) began a large-scale, long-term study that consisted of a set of clinical trials and an observational study, which together involved 161,808 "generally healthy" postmenopausal women aged 50 to 79 years. I put quotation marks around *generally healthy* because you'll see a little later that many of these women did have medical problems. The clinical trials were designed to test the effects of post-menopausal hormone therapy (HT), diet modification, and calcium and vitamin D supplements on heart disease, fractures, and breast and colorectal cancers.[1]

A lot of abbreviations are used to describe different hormone regimens, and as I mentioned earlier, they can have very different impacts. HT includes both Premarin and Prempro as well as any other estrogen alone or estrogen in combination with a progestogen. When estrogen is used alone, it is called estrogen therapy or ET; when estrogen is used together with a progestogen, it is called EPT. A major part of the confusion surrounding the WHI studies stems from the fact that the terms for these very different ways of giving estrogen are often used interchangeably. So whenever you read about risks and benefits of estrogen, be sure you understand what treatment the article is specifically referring to.

Abbreviations in *The Estrogen Fix*

ET	Estrogen therapy	Estrogen alone: either oral, via skin, or vaginal—replaces ERT
EPT	Estrogen-progestogen therapy	Estrogen plus a hormone that acts like progesterone
HT	Hormone therapy	Estrogen alone or combined with a progestogen (progestin or progesterone)—replaces HRT
HRT	Hormone replacement therapy	See HT
ERT	Estrogen replacement therapy	Replaced by ET
MPA	Medroxyprogesterone acetate	A synthetic progestogen, also called a progestin
MHT	Menopausal hormone therapy	See HT

The first published WHI study compared a placebo with Prempro, which combines the conjugated estrogen Premarin with the synthetic progesterone medroxyprogesterone acetate (MPA sold as Provera), the most commonly prescribed progestin at the time of the study. Women in this study had a uterus and required the progestin to prevent cancer of the lining of the uterus. The second study compared a placebo to the estrogen Premarin in women who had their uterus removed (hysterectomy) and did not require a progestogen. The WHI study was supposed to continue for 15 years.

On July 9, 2002, after approximately 5.2 years, the WHI issued a news release saying that the Prempro study would be stopped effective immediately, because the data to date showed a definite link between Prempro and an increased risk of breast cancer or suffering a heart attack, blood clots, or stroke. The results made front-page, above-the-fold headlines in newspapers and were the opening stories on evening news programs. The *New York Times* called the findings "A Shock to the Medical System." The *Washington Post* declared "A High Price for HT: No One Warned She Might Pay with Cancer."

By 2002, 40 percent of postmenopausal women in the United States were using HT to relieve the debilitating symptoms of menopause—night sweats, hot flashes, heart palpitations, and moodiness. Overnight, sales of premarin dropped 73 percent as thousands of doctors stopped prescribing estrogen—all kinds of estrogen and any medicine containing estrogen. Millions of women, who felt they had been duped and used as laboratory rats, instantly discontinued taking their estrogen-containing medicines. For those who insisted on continuing to use either Prempro or Premarin, many doctors required women to sign informed consents. Fear trumped reason, and front-page news affected doctors and their patients alike. Women and doctors had believed that estrogen was supposed to make women feel better without causing other medical issues; now doctors feared they had done their patients harm and patients believed they had been harmed.

It's difficult for many to remember or understand the panic that ensued when the WHI results were announced. To put it in historical perspective, just 10 months earlier America was attacked on September 11, 2001, and people were still feeling extremely vulnerable. When news of the canceled WHI study broke on July 9, 2002, many women felt as if they had been misled and were at risk of breast cancer, heart attack, and stroke. As many threw away their estrogen, anxiety levels skyrocketed.

I wish we could turn back the clock.

The 2002 WHI study contained a huge flaw that skewed the results and caused many women to forgo what we now know are the positive benefits of estrogen. I call these "estrogen myth-conceptions."

After practicing medicine for so many years and seeing the positive results of prescribing estrogen, I was skeptical about the findings and

SUSAN was 52 and had gone through surgical menopause at age 49 after her uterus and ovaries were removed. When she came to see me, she was still struggling with hot flashes, and vaginal dryness had become a problem for her, so she decided she wanted to try taking estrogen. She had not taken it earlier because she was afraid of the risks, and now that she was asking for it, her doctor recommended she not take it because she felt that Susan's hot flashes were likely to stop soon. But Susan was just 3 years into menopause and early in her estrogen window, which made her a good candidate to take estrogen. We discussed the symptoms she was having and the options available to treat them, and addressed her fears about taking estrogen. After our discussion, she started on an estrogen patch and is now symptom-free well within her estrogen window.

was reluctant to change my opinion based on just one study. I continued to prescribe Premarin to those women who wanted to continue with it and tried to switch patients from Prempro to Premarin or other estrogens plus a bioidentical progesterone. Remember, the information about side effects of the 2002 WHI study had to do with Prempro, which contained Provera; it was not specifically a report on Premarin or estrogen alone—except that Premarin is an estrogen and Prempro does contain Premarin. Unfortunately, all estrogen-containing medications were lumped together and perceived as one and the same. As you'll find out, they aren't.

I began taking a detailed look at the 2002 WHI study and how the news-making conclusions were reached. When I did, I was stunned to discover that the controversy surrounding taking estrogen was based on flawed study design and misinterpreted data. I then began to uncover the flaws within the WHI study.

Up to this date, all the data had been observational, meaning there were no controls for comparisons. This new WHI study pulled the rug out from under all the previously published observations about estrogen. Not only had estrogen been perceived as safe and beneficial, but it was also used as a treatment for advanced breast cancer. This new idea that estrogen was bad and caused breast cancer, among other things, was a total reversal of the existing medical beliefs at that time.

I read and reread the study and its conclusions, spoke with leading doctors and researchers in the fields of women's health and menopause, and studied each new article that came out from the WHI and related sources. Remember that in 2004, just 2 years later, the estrogen-only arm of the WHI study did not show the same negative results; Premarin alone did not cause an increase in breast cancer or heart disease. So there were reasons to question the validity of the 2002 findings. A number of prominent doctors, including Wulf H. Utian, MD, who founded the North American Menopause Society, and Philip Sarrel, MD, of Yale University, didn't accept the study's findings as gospel, but evidence was necessary to prove that the results were wrong. The 2002 WHI study collected data in a quality way, but the big flaw was in the study design, and that caused incorrect interpretation of the information.

I owed it to my wife, Sharon, and my patients to learn everything about the topic, so they wouldn't have to choose between no treatment and treatment that they believed would alleviate their menopause symptoms but perhaps also increase their risk of death. Why should midlife women have to "tough it out" and suffer from their menopausal symptoms or live symptom-free and filled with fear and anxiety just because one study made claims unsubstantiated elsewhere?

My impression was that since participants in the 2004 study took estrogen only, and participants in both the 2002 and the 2004 studies received the same dosages of Premarin, the variable had to be Provera. Provera is known to narrow blood vessels and to undo the benefits of estrogen, which is part of the reason why I earlier referred to Provera as the bad guy. At that point I immediately stopped prescribing Provera, which was the progestogen combined with Premarin, and shifted my patients to bioidentical progesterone (see page 57).

I also noticed differences in the outcomes of the women in the two studies: The women in the 2004 Premarin-only study were also between the ages of 50 and 79, but when the study was stopped roughly 7 years after it began, those same women showed no increased risk of cardiovascular heart disease or heart attack and appeared to have *less* risk of breast cancer. For another 7 years there would not be enough numbers to prove that estrogen only lowered the risk of breast cancer.[2]

I saw a story beginning to take shape, but it would take me nearly a decade until further analysis of the same data and newer studies could prove that a woman's age and the number of years since she entered menopause play a major role when it comes to the risks and benefits of estrogen.

Prior to the first WHI study's findings in 2002, estrogen was thought to be a fountain of youth. Suddenly it was considered a risk factor for death and disease. As the study's flaws were being pointed out, the same doctors who once thought estrogen provided only positive benefits either didn't realize it or didn't want to go out on a limb and say they had it wrong yet again. I can appreciate how they felt, but not focusing on the facts would cause millions of women to continue not receiving estrogen, and I didn't want that to happen to them or to my wife.

I realized that the majority of women can safely take estrogen for effective relief of their menopausal symptoms starting at a certain time in their lives without having to worry about an increased risk of cancer, heart disease, or other illnesses later. How? First, by revisiting the previous data, asking the right questions, and coming up with appropriate answers. Second, by publishing new studies that are better designed to ask the right question: When Premarin (estrogen only) or Prempro (estrogen plus progestogen) is given to a group of younger women and compared to women of similar age and medical histories who don't take these hormones, does estrogen offer benefits?

The answer is yes, particularly for the estrogen-only group. I can now confidently offer my patients estrogen and its many benefits. I can allay their fears by clarifying the misinformation published and publicized in 2002. Many of my patients are taking estrogen at the opportune time in life with great success. And there is plenty of evidence that you can too!

Unfortunately, today's media have been exceptionally silent about the subsequent reversal of thinking during the last several years as the results of better-designed estrogen studies have appeared. And to be fair, these new findings are also hard to believe because estrogen's dangers have become so ingrained in the minds of many. Again, here is the contrast: It's like a correction in the newspaper that is buried with other emendations and never receives the same attention as the error-filled story. This new information has largely gone unreported yet has remained hidden in clear view, which means that millions of women are suffering unnecessarily and jeopardizing their long-term health. Fortunately, organizations like the American College of Obstetricians and Gynecologists (ACOG), the North American Menopause Society (NAMS), the American Society for Reproductive Medicine (ASRM), and Advancing Health After Hysterectomy (Ahah) are also working to raise awareness of this issue.

Deciding whether or not to take estrogen is crucial for women today. In 1900 the average life span for a woman was 48 years, so not many women had to worry about menopause. Today is different. We live in a time when the average woman's life span is an astonishing 81 years and becoming longer every year. Questions about how to deal with menopause and the years beyond have become more frequent, more pressing, and much more relevant. A recent study showed that the number of women living to be 100 increased by 50 percent between 1990 and 2013,[3] but they have a number of health conditions. As more women (and men) are living longer, enabling women to begin taking estrogen during their estrogen window will help them reach old age with fewer serious medical conditions and eliminate many menopause symptoms along the way. This is the basis of the estrogen fix.

The History of Hormone Therapy

When the FDA approved the estrogen Premarin in 1942, for the first time, doctors immediately began to prescribe it to women to relieve their hot flashes and other symptoms of menopause. The estrogen revolution gained momentum in the 1950s, and in the 1960s estrogen's popularity continued to grow. To spread the word farther and faster, Wyeth-Ayerst Laboratories hired Brooklyn gynecologist Robert Wilson in 1966 to author *Feminine Forever* and extol the virtues of estrogen, even calling it a "fountain of youth" that would prevent the inevitable "living decay" of menopause.

By the late 1960s, Premarin was the most frequently prescribed drug in the United States.[4] Everyone wanted to take estrogen. For a while, it was even prescribed to men, but the results for men were harmful and sometimes fatal. And while everyone was seeking this "fountain of youth," no one had yet discovered the optimum safe dosage required to do the job without unnecessary risk, what age to start taking it, or the length of time a woman should stay on the hormone. There was a growing understanding of the importance of taking a progestogen to protect the uterine lining—after long periods of estrogen alone, women would develop a precancerous tissue buildup called hyperplasia and a subset of those women would develop cancer of the uterine lining—but initially, the only commercially available progestogen was Provera. Provera had a number of worrisome side effects, including a possible increased risk of breast cancer, and it was not FDA approved for preventing uterine hyperplasia, so doctors weren't prescribing it along with Premarin. For these reasons, throughout much of this time, estrogen was given alone.

In 1975 and 1976 a series of three articles from three different centers were published in the *New England Journal of Medicine* that proved estrogen alone given to women with a uterus for long periods of time caused uterine cancer.[5, 6, 7] Public opinion immediately turned against estrogen, and its popularity tumbled.

In the 1980s evidence was growing that estrogen was helpful in preventing heart attacks in women. The belief that estrogen was cardioprotective was so strong that gynecologists and primary-care providers prescribed it not only to *treat* symptoms of menopause but also to *prevent* heart disease. Unfortunately, this information was based on observational studies, meaning they were not randomized with half of the women taking estrogen and the other half a placebo.

So to find out how estrogen might help prevent heart disease, a randomized study called the PEPI (Postmenopausal Estrogen/Progestin Interventions) Trial was established and included Premarin plus Provera.[8] A total of 875 women were studied for 3 years. When the results were published in 1995, Premarin plus Provera was found to have a positive effect on HDL or good cholesterol, and it protected the uterine lining cells from cancer. Following the PEPI Trial, the FDA approved Provera to prevent cancer of the uterine lining in postmenopausal women, and Provera became the most widely used progestogen for this purpose. Many unanswered questions remained, which is how Provera came to be tested in the WHI studies.

In the 1990s the WHI was created. Two different initial studies for two different groups of women with two different treatments were designed to last 15 years. Group one included 16,608 women who had a uterus, and they received either Prempro or a placebo. Group two included 10,739 women who did not have a uterus because of hysterectomy, and they received either Premarin or a placebo. These studies were the first multiyear, large-scale randomized clinical trials to determine the risks and benefits of these two types of medication on two groups of women. Premarin was still one of the most popular medications in the United States, as was Prempro, since Provera was now an FDA-approved medication to prevent cancer of the uterine lining.

In 2002 the first WHI study was abruptly shut down early at the 5.2 years mark after preliminary data indicated a small, measured increase in risk of breast cancer and cardiovascular heart disease among women who took Prempro. Since this was a prevention study, any increased health risk required that it immediately be discontinued. You can imagine that when the NIH shuts down a study and it becomes front-page news that suggests the medicine you are taking causes breast cancer and heart disease, you would panic if you were taking that medication. And panic causes lower objectivity. No one took the time to read the fine print.

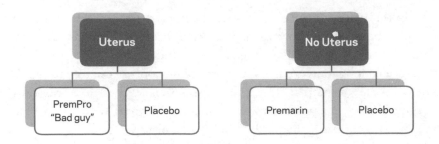

The WHI studies had a "fatal" flaw. Instead of comparing apples with apples, they compared apples with oranges. They compared a placebo group of mostly younger women (mostly 50 to 59 years old) to a study group of mostly (75 percent) older women (mostly 60 to 79 years old). And to make matters worse, more than 60 percent of the women in the older group were lifelong smokers; many had some form of heart disease and were overweight. Many in the older group also had diabetes and high blood pressure. It's no surprise that older women with more medical problems would have poorer outcomes—and they did.

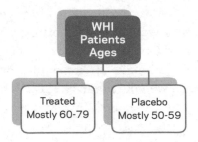

Yet when the NIH released the 2002 WHI results, the risks were placed solely at the feet of the Prempro, which, as you'll discover, did play a role; but the study did not consider preexisting risk factors or how much time had passed since each woman entered menopause. "Estrogen" was blamed entirely as the culprit. It was like comparing car death statistics between drunk or sleep-impaired drivers and those who were sober and rested. You don't have to be a research scientist to know that this was poor science and poor analysis of the information. As mentioned, since this was a prevention study, any reported increase in risk meant the study had to be discontinued immediately.

The researchers running the study knew the women taking Prempro were not comparable with the women in the control group because of the significant differences in age, but they didn't know how to overcome this hurdle. When the researchers first started recruiting subjects for the study in September 1993, so many menopausal women were already taking Premarin or Prempro, they had difficulty finding age-matched women for the control group who *weren't* taking it.

Instead they put together a group of women who were mostly aged 60 and over, all of whom were no longer taking Premarin or Prempro. But many of these women were heavy smokers and had poor heart health, diabetes, or high blood pressure. Yet amazingly, all that crucial health information and their age differences were overlooked and under-reported when the WHI researchers wrote their conclusions about the safety and efficacy of Prempro. Many years later, these poorly analyzed, incorrectly interpreted data remain the basis of the misgivings and fears attached to estrogen. The patients who come to see me today as they enter menopause are still talking about those erroneous conclusions. I hear over and over again from these women that they feel they have no choice but to tough out their menopausal symptoms. It's as though taking any form of estrogen would be causing them early death. Almost every woman I see fears taking estrogen because of the outdated and incorrect WHI information. Once I explain the facts and reassure them, they become eager to discover their estrogen window.

A Menopause Breakthrough

The confusion from the WHI study left me wondering what other studies, clinical trials, and information revealed about the positive versus negative effects of estrogen. I started reading all the estrogen information I could find to understand why estrogen continued to be the 800-pound gorilla in the room for menopause, women, and their doctors. I analyzed years of data, poring over major and minor studies and hundreds of peer-reviewed journal articles and papers presented at meetings and symposia. I interviewed fellow experienced doctors and top researchers, including Drs. Pauline Maki, Phil Sarrel, Wulf Utian, Isaac Schiff, Mary Jane Minkin, JoAnn V. Pinkerton, JoAnn E. Manson, James A. Simon, Sara Gottfried, Andrew Kaunitz, and others as editor of *The Hot Years-My Menopause Magazine*.

I did this because menopause is one of the most challenging periods in a woman's life. As an ob-gyn and menopause expert, I witness on an almost-daily basis how menopause symptoms affect the quality of my patients' lives and their performance in the workplace. Surely there had to be some evidence-based way that estrogen could be used to bring relief.

Each article, presentation, and interview contained a golden nugget of information that together created a pot of gold—something really valuable to help Sharon, my patients, and women everywhere. I came to realize there is such a thing I call the estrogen window, the time in a woman's life when she can most safely take estrogen and benefit from it in many ways.

Consider the hormone insulin for a diabetic patient. Taken at the right time, insulin regulates blood sugar, keeps diabetes under control, and wards off potentially devastating side effects. If insulin is given at the wrong time, a diabetic can go into diabetic shock. For estrogen, too, timing is very important. As a medication, it is not about being either good or bad. It's all about the timing. If taken at the right time, estrogen provides dramatic relief for the most troubling menopausal symptoms while at the same time providing a host of benefits, including:

- Extended protection from heart attacks and heart failure
- Reduced risk of Alzheimer's disease and other forms of cognitive decline
- Reduced risk of osteoporosis
- Beneficial cosmetic effects on the structure and resiliency of the skin
- Relief of sexual problems such as vaginal dryness and painful intercourse
- Relief from troubling and sometimes disabling hot flashes
- Improved quality of sleep
- Stabilized mood, particularly in women who have a known mental health diagnosis
- Lowered risk of type 2 diabetes
- Support for bladder tissue and lower risk of recurring urinary tract infections

Taken during a woman's estrogen window, estrogen accomplishes all these astonishing feats with minimal increased health risks. How long her estrogen window stays open depends on two things: which estrogen-containing medicine is used and which symptom or condition is being targeted, which I explain throughout *The Estrogen Fix*.

If the same woman takes the same drug after her estrogen window has closed, there may be an increased risk of serious side effects. Her odds for developing cardiovascular disease, blood clots, cancer, and cognitive decline become higher. But remember: It's not the estrogen that is bad; it's the Provera combined with the estrogen and *when* it is taken during a woman's life, or the timing, that are bad.

Too many women believe they have to struggle through this phase of life without assistance, and somehow if they do that and forgo estrogen, they will come out on the other side without any consequences. Others think that if they take estrogen and get almost immediate symptom relief, they will be diagnosed with breast cancer or heart disease a few years down the road. Nothing could be further from the truth. *The Estrogen Fix* will help you "figure it out" so you won't have to "tough it out."

It's ironic that the treatment women have avoided because they fear increased odds of developing a dreaded disease is in fact the very treatment that can offer greatly expanded protection *against* developing those same potentially deadly conditions *after* menopause. The key to using estrogen successfully is to take the right estrogen and to take it at the right time for at least 5 to 7 years following the onset of menopause.

It has taken decades to undo the damage done by one flawed study and change people's minds, even doctors', despite efforts from members of NAMS, ASRM, and ACOG. On June 3, 2015, NAMS[9] issued a statement and editorial on hormone therapy in women *after* age 65 that says:

- HT is the most effective treatment for symptoms of menopause.

- Vasomotor symptoms [hot flashes] may persist for more than a decade in many women and may continue in women after the age of 65, and these symptoms can disrupt sleep and adversely affect health and quality of life.

- Provided a woman has been advised of increased risks associated with continuing HT beyond age 60 and she has appropriate medical supervision, extending use of HT with the lowest effective dose is acceptable under some circumstances in women older than 65.

●Use of HT should be individualized and not discontinued based solely on a woman's age.

On October 6, 2016, at the NAMS Annual Scientific Meeting, Executive Director JoAnn V. Pinkerton, MD, revealed their latest position statement about HT, which represents a consensus of over 20 international experts.[10]

The bottom line: Overall, HT has clear benefits for the treatment of hot flashes and bone loss prevention. These benefits are most favorable among women aged younger than 60 years who are within 10 years of menopause onset and have no medical reasons they can't take HT. Women older than age 60 who begin HT beyond 10 years of menopause onset appear to have a less favorable benefit-risk ratio because of elevated risks of coronary heart disease, stroke, venous thromboembolism, and dementia—i.e., it's all about the estrogen window.

The science is clear: Based on clinical studies that have appeared in multiple peer-reviewed medical journals, estrogen *can* be taken safely if used in the right way at the right time for the right length of time.

If you're like my patients, you probably have a lot of questions: Is estrogen really as safe as you say? Do I take pills, use a cream, or apply a patch? What's the right dosage for me? When should I start? How do I know when to stop? Which estrogen should I take? Which progestogen should I take? All your questions will be answered in *The Estrogen Fix,* so you'll be prepared to have an informed conversation with your physician or health-care provider.

Chapter 2

Estrogen and You

W hen you think about being a woman, what comes to mind? When I asked my 93-year-old mother, she immediately said, "soft and gentle, womanhood, become old enough to get married and have a family, love, tenderness, and understanding." Then she said, "As a little girl, I used to sing the nursery rhyme 'Girls are made of sugar and spice and everything nice.'"

If a reproductive endocrinologist had written that rhyme, I'm sure the sugar and spice would have included a splash of estrogen. Puberty. Menstruation. Pregnancy. Perimenopause. Menopause. All these changes involve estrogen. Let's time travel through a woman's life and examine each of these biological transitions and the role that estrogen plays in them. This journey will help you understand what is happening to your body and how this eventually ties into menopause and your estrogen window.

Puberty marks the awakening of hormones and signals the beginning of fertility in girls and boys. It is a time of development—generally between 10 to 13 years of age for girls, 11 to 14 for boys—when a child's body turns into an adult's. Everyone is born producing some estrogen; but when girls enter puberty, their ovaries begin to produce significantly more of it. (Boys entering puberty produce more of the hormone testosterone.) The outpouring of estrogen and androgens during puberty causes significant physical and emotional changes. Girls develop breasts, body hair grows in the armpits and pubic area, hips and butts become curvier, hair on legs and arms becomes darker, body odors are more noticeable, acne may develop as a result of oilier skin, mood swings occur, and thoughts of romance and sexual attractions are frequent. It's also the beginning of menstruation.

Menstruation, or menses, is the monthly shedding of the lining of the uterus. Once menstruation begins, it signals puberty[1] and the beginning of reproductive life. Initially, menses are usually very irregular because of fluctuating hormone levels. This fluctuation has a major impact on mood that usually evens out. Since menstruation usually occurs every 21 to 35 days for 2 to 7 days, it is commonly referred to as a period. The first period a young woman has is called menarche; it usually occurs between the ages of 10 and 14—sometimes earlier, sometimes later. It's important to remember at what age your first period occurred for your medical history. Women who began their periods before age 12 have about 20 percent higher breast and uterine cancer risks compared to those who began their periods after age 14.[2, 3]

A woman can expect to menstruate from about ages 12½ to 51, roughly 35 to 40 years. During that time her ovaries have a reservoir of eggs, and some will be released each month throughout her reproductive years to make pregnancy possible. Women usually stop menstruating when they are pregnant or breastfeeding, but during that time their ovaries continue to produce eggs each month, so it doesn't change the onset of menopause, when the last egg has been released. The dwindling number of eggs ushers in irregular hormones and perimenopause.

Perimenopause literally means "around menopause" and refers to the months and years (up to 10) leading up to the last menstrual period plus 1 year after the last menstrual period, which defines menopause. Because the symptoms are most intense in the last 2 years of perimenopause, some women think they are in menopause, although they still are having irregular periods.

Perimenopause is a time of widely fluctuating hormones and the stage when a woman's menstrual cycle begins to change and become more and more irregular. Estrogen and progesterone transition from balanced and synchronized to unbalanced and unsynchronized. Because the ovaries contain fewer eggs, they become more resistant to ovulation, which means releasing an egg, so the pituitary gland's follicle-stimulating hormone (FSH) increases in an attempt to motivate the ovaries to release an egg. Increasing FSH levels determined by a blood test suggest that a woman is in perimenopause.

In 2012 a group of researchers from five countries and multiple disciplines reviewed all the blood tests and markers and symptoms of menopause studies from around the world and came to an agreement on how to define perimenopause. The large study was called STRAW (Stages of Reproductive Aging Workshop).[4] The researchers couldn't make sense of the information when they tried to define menopause and perimenopause symptoms by age. But when they looked at the onset of menopause as time "0" and then counted both forward and backward by years, suddenly the information lined up. Perimenopause is defined in that study as the 2 years leading up to menopause, and menopause is defined as 1 year after the last menstrual period. As you will discover in the chapters to come, it's the onset of menopause and not age that will define the opening of your estrogen window.

Perhaps you're hot one minute then pulling on a sweater the next because you're chilled. Maybe your thinking is a bit foggy and your mind doesn't seem as sharp as it once was or all your pants are suddenly feeling a size too small. Do you have heart palpitations? Not interested in sex? Do you urinate more frequently than you used to? Are you 50 years old, give or take a few years? There's probably nothing "wrong" with you. Your body is transitioning toward menopause.

Common Perimenopause Symptoms

- Acne
- Anxiety
- Bloating
- Breast tenderness
- Crying
- Decreased libido
- Facial hair
- Forgetfulness
- Frequent need to urinate
- Hair loss or thinning

- Headaches
- Hot flashes
- Interrupted sleep
- Irregular periods
- Mood swings
- Night sweats
- Urinary incontinence
- Vaginal dryness
- Weight gain, especially around the middle

Menarche → | **FMP (0)** →

Stage	-5	-4	-3b	-3a	-2	-1	+1a	+1b	+1c	+2
Terminology	REPRODUCTIVE				MENOPAUSAL TRANSITION		POSTMENOPAUSE			
	Early	Peak	Late		Early	Late	Early			Late
					Perimenopause					
Duration					Variable	1–3 years	2 years (1 + 1)		3–6 years	Remaining lifespan
PRINCIPAL CRITERIA										
Menstrual cycle	Variable to regular	Regular	Regular	Subtle changes in flow/length	Variable length Persistent ≥7-day difference in length of consecutive cycles	Interval of amenorrhea of ≥60 days				
SUPPORTIVE CRITERIA										
Endocrine										
FSH			Low	Variable*	↑ Variable	↑ >25 IU/L**	Stabilizes			
AMH			Low	Low	Low	Low	Very low			
Inhibin B				Low	Low	Low	Very low			
Antral Follicle Count			Low	Low	Low	Very low	Very low			
DESCRIPTIVE CHARACTERISTICS										
Symptoms					Vasomotor symptoms Likely	Vasomotor symptoms Very likely				Increasing symptoms of urogenital atrophy

* Blood draw on cycle days 2–5.
** Approximate expected level based on assays using current international pituitary standard.[5]
↑ = Elevated
Menarche = first menstrual period
FMP = final menstrual period[5]

Most young girls have the "talk" with their mothers or other women about menstruation, sex, and having babies. When a girl gets her period, she learns that she's fertile and can expect to menstruate every month. On the other end of the age spectrum, women typically don't have the "talk" with their mothers about menopause and aren't taught what to expect. And your experience can be very different from those of your friends—either much easier or much more challenging. For most, perimenopause comes on slowly and without much notice. You have an occasional heart palpitation. You find that it takes you longer to become sexually aroused. You've added a few pounds around the middle. Over time, more symptoms crop up, intensify, and become one perfect storm.

For many women, perimenopause and menopause are synonymous with getting old. Just saying it carries a negative burden. The good news is, the more you understand your estrogen window, the more you will be able to put things in perspective and gain control over your symptoms. That will make you feel both healthier and happier. Another good thing is that most women only get some of the symptoms—almost no one gets them all.

"What is happening to my body and my brain?" Are you a woman who is used to juggling work, social, and family obligations and who once slept through the night and managed your days? Now, do you suddenly find yourself waking up at 4:00 a.m. with heart palpitations or feeling sleepy, anxious, or teary during the day? Do you sometimes lose focus and have a shorter fuse than you used to? Throw in a few mood swings, headaches, and forgetting where the car is parked and you begin to wonder if something is physically or mentally wrong with you.

Hormonally, perimenopause looks like going through puberty backward, and it brings with it some of the same experiences. During perimenopause, shifting production levels of the hormones estrogen and progesterone cause periods to become irregular and vary in the amount of flow. A woman may have regular periods for 3 months, then none for 6, then periods that arrive regularly for several months, or periods for 6 months, none for 4, then heavy flow or light spotting in-between, and so on. The variables all depend on the individual woman. For the majority of women, perimenopause occurs during their forties, but like everything else on this journey, it may occur earlier or later.

The average length of perimenopause, and the most intense symptoms, lasts for 4 years, but again, since everyone is different, that too can vary. Some women have symptoms for 10 years. Occasionally symptoms will last longer. Over time, estrogen levels will drop to prepuberty levels, periods stop entirely, and it is no longer possible to become pregnant. During perimenopause, estrogen levels plunge and soar like a wild hormonal roller-coaster ride. Instead of estrogen and progesterone levels working together with precision, they work somewhat independently. Progesterone levels don't typically rise unless the ovary ovulates an egg. Progesterone's primary role is to stabilize the uterine lining so an embryo can implant (the word *progesterone* stems from "pro-gestation"), but progesterone also plays a role in a woman's moods by attaching to the same sites in the brain as the neurochemical GABA, a hormone that helps reduce anxiety. Lower progesterone levels affect women differently, but persistently low levels are believed to play a major role in the mood changes and swings so often experienced by women during perimenopause and menopause.

As uncomfortable and as aggravating as perimenopause can be, know that, like puberty, it is only temporary and will end. The meno-

---

Perimenopause Testing

Your doctor may order an FSH blood test to see if you are in perimenopause. Values above 11 mIU/mL may suggest early perimenopause and values above 20 mIU/mL clearly identify perimenopause. Another test that can be ordered is called anti-Müllerian hormone or AMH. For this test, the lower the value, the closer to menopause, although the FSH test is not well suited to telling you how close. In a well-done study from the University of Pennsylvania,[6] an AMH level below 0.20 ng/mL suggested that the median time to menopause was 5.99 years for women aged 45 to 48 and 9.94 years for women in the 35 to 39 age group. With AMH levels above 1.50 ng/mL, the median time to menopause was 6.23 years in the older group and more than 13 years in the youngest age group. Smoking significantly reduced the time to menopause.

To discover how your perimenopause experience compares to other women, take this free 2-minute quiz at MenopauseQuiz.com.

pausal transition symptoms typically decline significantly 2 years after your last menstrual period, which is 1 year after menopause begins.

Menopause is the last hormonal transition phase. The zigzagging estrogen and progesterone levels I mentioned earlier continue to trend downward until they reach very low baseline levels. There are no longer any eggs within the ovaries (or no ovaries because of surgery), or the ovaries contain eggs but they no longer respond to FSH. In either instance, FSH levels remain constantly elevated, usually above 40 mIU/mL. The medical definition of menopause is for a woman to go 1 year without a period, which typically occurs when she is in her late forties or early fifties in Western countries.

ONSET OF MENOPAUSE	FREQUENCY
Before age 20	1 out of 10,000 women
Before age 30	1 out of 1,000 women
Before age 40	1 out of 100 women
Before age 45	1 out of 10–20 women

Compiled by Mache Seibel, MD

Menopause can take place in one of the three following ways:

1. Natural or spontaneous menopause: When a woman's ovaries naturally stop making enough estrogen to produce a menstrual cycle.

2. Surgical menopause: When a woman's ovaries are removed by surgery prior to natural menopause. The woman is in menopause from the time the ovaries are removed. If the ovaries are removed before age 46, the woman is in early menopause. Having a hysterectomy (surgical removal of the uterus) will stop menstruation, but it does not cause menopause unless both ovaries are removed, which is called a bilateral oophorectomy. It's important to know that if you have a hysterectomy, even if your ovaries are left in, you will most likely lose some of your ovaries' hormone-producing ability within the first few years after surgery. This will be discussed later.

3. Induced or iatrogenic menopause: When a woman's ovaries cease to function because of radiation treatments, chemotherapy, or the use of some other drugs.

LISA SASEVICH received the Distinguished Mentor Award from the Business Expert Forum at the Harvard Faculty Club. She has also received the coveted eWomenNetwork Foundation Champion award for her generous fundraising and ranked on the prestigious Inc. 500/5000 list of America's fastest-growing private companies for 2 years in a row.

DR. MACHE SEIBEL: Lisa, you are a successful businesswoman who has helped thousands of women reach their potential. Can you share your thoughts about women in the workplace and menopause? What can women can do to balance work and life?

LISA SASEVICH: I believe that when women are in their forties, intelligence and life experience come together. This is a magical time for women to step up and own who they are in the world. Too often, they're trying to do everything right, but something is going wrong and they can't figure out what the problem is.

MS: One woman told me she would rather be on national television and say she got fired than to say she had a hot flash. How can we normalize the experiences that women go through naturally as something that's just part of the course of life? What can you say to women who may be at this time of life to help them?

LS: When I gave birth to my children, I was in my mid- and late thirties, very close to 40. When friends close to my age were also pregnant, they didn't tell anyone until they were past the first trimester. I never understood that. I wanted the support and the sharing, so I've always been someone who is a little more forthcoming about the personal things going on in my life. When I'm standing on a stage and giving a presentation, I know that if I suddenly have a hot flash, others in the room are going through the same thing. The more open we can be about our discoveries and our journeys, the more other women will reflect on their own discoveries and journeys.

MS: You're saying to use these opportunities to get support as opposed to feeling isolated.

LS: Yes! That's my philosophy, and it works well for me. When it comes to menopause, you are neither the first person nor the only person to go through it, and there's no reason to suffer in silence.

There's so much women can do in the 10 years before menopause. If I had waited until that time, I would have missed situations that would have affected my longevity and my clarity of thinking, which is important to me. So by being open, I was able to attract the right kind of advice.

MS: Do you talk to women who are unaware or unwilling to admit that they are going through a new phase in life? "What happened? My energy is gone. My thinking is gone."

LS: One woman in her midforties invested in our program at the highest level, a six-figure investment, and took 24-hour flights to attend our meetings. She took my systems, spoke all over the world, and transitioned into doing teleseminars and webinars so she could do more business at home and be with family. After 6 months, she came to a meeting and couldn't stop crying. Here was a woman who had been on top of the world and sought after in her industry, but somehow had lost her motivation. She wasn't sleeping well. She was an emotional wreck. She considered giving up her business. Hundreds of other people were sitting there and trying to coach her on her mind-set and help her with team structures and sales structures, but every suggestion and idea fell flat. Suddenly, another woman said to her, "Have you had your hormone levels checked? When's the last time you had a physical with your doctor?"

She saw her doctor, and within a month, she was the entrepreneurial rock star I once knew. It was like night and day! She started estrogen therapy and was back on track with her business and her marriage, which had been affected as well.

MS: Often perimenopause suddenly causes your clarity to be affected, your energy levels to become low, and your moods to go up and down like a seesaw, but it's difficult to see these changes in yourself. Sometimes someone else has to point out that perhaps you're transitioning to or already in menopause, especially if you are younger. You're saying acknowledge what you're feeling and seek some help.

LS: Absolutely! This is the most magical time of your life, and if you're not feeling like yourself, be proactive and serious about finding out if you are heading toward menopause and what to do

(continued)

about it. The great news is that it's not as complicated as you might think.

MS: There's a lot of fear when it comes to menopause, because it's so unfamiliar, but it doesn't have to be that way. Women are so important to our society and to our family system. Women make 85 percent of the purchases and health-care decisions in their families. These are huge responsibilities while also nurturing their kids, their partners, and their aging parents, and all while working. Too often I find that women don't take the time to nurture themselves. You're suggesting that women be open to relying on other women for information and insight during this time of life.

LS: Even if you're 10 years before you'll enter menopause, I encourage you to learn about your estrogen window, which I learned about from you. If you're not feeling like yourself, is it work or family related? Physical? Psychological? Or the one that a lot of us forget to look at—hormonal?

MS: Do you have any other tips for women as they transition through this time of life?

LS: First, realize that there are no second chances in life. It's amazing how fast time goes by, especially as we get older. Life is not a dress rehearsal; you get one shot. This is it; you don't know how long you have. If you're feeling off, get on it.

What Is Estrogen?

Estrogen is a steroid hormone that conjures up "all things female": curvy bodies, breasts, ovaries—the stuff that turns a girl into a woman. While everyone is born producing some natural estrogen, when a girl enters puberty and throughout her reproductive years, estrogen levels are much higher. Chemically, estrogen is an arrangement of four chemical rings joined together that look like chicken wire.

Hormones are in a class of what's called signaling molecules because they are produced by an endocrine gland in one part of the body that communicates with, or "signals," various other parts of the body to accomplish specific tasks, such as regulating bone health, boosting the body's immunity, or influencing the timing of a woman's monthly cycle. They regulate how our bodies function and how we think and behave.

A woman's body makes three different forms of estrogen. They are estrone (E1), estradiol (E2), and estriol (E3). E1 is made in many tissues, especially fat. E1 is made in much higher quantities in obese women, which is one of the reasons why heavier women are more prone to gallstones and uterine cancer. E2 is largely produced in the ovaries. E3 is produced from the placenta during pregnancy.

THE THREE BIOIDENTICAL ESTROGENS

E1 Estrone

E2 Estradiol, 17β-estradiol

E3 Estriol

These three hormones are the estrogens called bioidentical, no matter what type of pharmacy you buy them in. And no matter where you buy them they are not natural and are not naturally occurring in plants; they must be manufactured from compounds found in plants such as soybeans and wild yams. Humans don't have the needed enzymes to turn plant compounds into bioidentical hormones. But once manufactured, they are bioidentical; they have the chemical structure identical to what the body makes naturally. These estrogens play different roles at different times in a woman's reproductive life. *Bioidentical* is not a scientific term. Dr. Wulf Utian, founder of the North American Menopause Society, advocates that the correct term should be *compounded hormone therapy* (C-HT) if it is provided from a compounded pharmacy and *government-approved hormone therapy* if it is FDA approved from a traditional pharmacy. C-HT is not FDA approved.

Most of a woman's estradiol is made in her ovaries, although some is produced in other tissue, such as the adrenal glands. The ovaries also make estrone, but most estrone is manufactured primarily in the body's fat cells by a process called aromatization. The enzyme aromatase takes androgen (see "Other Hormones and Menopause" on page 29) hormones and aromatizes or converts them into estrone. Just as you might guess, women who have more fat on their bodies make more estrone. More estrone is good news for some women because it may lower their symptoms of menopause. But too much estrone is also a major reason why women who are significantly overweight have a higher risk of uterine cancer—three times higher if they are 25 to 50 pounds overweight and nine times higher if they are more than 50 pounds overweight. At the opposite extreme, women who are too thin and who have too little fat on their bodies may stop having periods altogether because their bodies don't produce enough estrogen.

Estradiol is the major estrogen produced by the ovaries before menopause. It is also the most potent—12 times more than estrone and 80 times more than estriol. After menopause, estradiol levels drop by as much as 90 percent because almost all of it comes from the ovaries, and they stop making it. Estrone levels drop by as much as one-third as the ovaries stop making it. But estrone does continue to be made in the body's fat tissue, and obese women (more than 20 percent over ideal body weight) can make up to 40 percent more estrone than non-obese women. Other organs, including the brain, muscles, lungs, skin, and bone marrow can also convert androgens (male hormones) into estrone. The body makes only very small amounts of estriol except during pregnancy, when the placenta increases production of the hormone by more than a thousandfold. In contrast to estradiol and estrone, estriol does not appear to be linked with any increased risk of cancer, but this hasn't been proven because enough studies haven't been done.

The point of this information is that estrogen is a very important hormone for women that affects almost every part of their bodies. Estrogen levels fluctuate each month and in each phase of a woman's life. When levels fluctuate, changes can be significant, and potentially affect all parts of the body. In perimenopause, hormonal fluctuations become very pronounced, sort of like they were in puberty, only in reverse order. And the impact on a woman's body from top to bottom can be equally profound.

And then comes menopause, with estrogen levels at only 10 percent of what they were at the peak of a woman's reproductive years. Now it's easy to understand how the many symptoms of menopause can slowly and steadily become part of a woman's life.

Other Hormones and Menopause

Testosterone and androstenedione (AN-drow–steen–DIE–own) are two androgen, or "male," hormones that also change during and after menopause. Although both men and women produce androgens, women have lower levels of them just like men have lower levels of estrogen than women. After menopause, testosterone levels drop by as much as 28 percent in women. Much of this drop is due to decreased testosterone production in the ovaries.

About 600,000 hysterectomies are performed annually in the United States. Many times a doctor may recommend taking out the ovaries at the same time to reduce the risk of ovarian cancer. If that happens, you will be in surgical menopause and a candidate for taking estrogen.

But what happens to your ovarian hormone levels if you have a hysterectomy and your ovaries are not removed? It would seem that if the ovaries were not removed, they would continue to work just like they did before the hysterectomy. But this is not the case. Many women who have hysterectomies go through a type of delayed surgical menopause. Women who have a total abdominal hysterectomy (TAH—meaning their uterus is removed through an abdominal incision but their ovaries are not) go through menopause an average of 5 years earlier than women who have not had a TAH.[7] Within the first 6 months after surgery, 25 percent lose ovarian function and within 3 years, 40 percent lose ovarian function. The average time an ovary continues to function after hysterectomy is 7 years. Indirectly, a hysterectomy without removing the ovaries can cause surgical menopause.

Why does this happen? When bloodflow to the ovaries is measured by special testing at the time of TAH, bloodflow is decreased by 80 percent.[8] That decrease in bloodflow causes ovarian tissue death, which is called infarction, much like a reduction in bloodflow to the heart causes a myocardial infarction, or heart attack. Even though the ovaries look normal at the time of surgery, a study done 1 year later showed the ovaries from all women who had a TAH had some area of infarction and accelerated loss of the number of eggs.[9, 10] This is important information for all women undergoing a hysterectomy to know and discuss with their doctor. If you have a hysterectomy when you are young, particularly age 44 or younger,[11] you may go into early menopause even if your ovaries are not removed, which is important to know because most hysterectomies are done in women before they enter menopause.

Hysterectomy Rates per 1,000 Women in the United States[12]

AGE RANGE	HYSTERECTOMIES/1,000 WOMEN
45–49	9.7
40–45	9.6
35–39	6.5
50–54	5.6

The average age for a hysterectomy is 46.1 years. By age 54, one-third of all women will have had a hysterectomy. Most of those women who have a hysterectomy before age 46 will have gone through early menopause. One of my patients, Sandra, was taken aback by her symptoms and said, "I can't be going through menopause; I still have my ovaries." This information can help a woman decide whether to have her ovaries removed if she is at significant risk of ovarian cancer; if she does not have her ovaries removed, she can have her FSH and estrogen levels followed in the months and years to come to see if she is going into early menopause.

After menopause, the adrenal glands slowly begin to produce lesser amounts of another hormone—androstenedione. Because the testosterone and androstenedione drop slowly, postmenopausal women who experience natural menopause often don't have a loss of libido. If there is a loss of libido and testosterone isn't low, taking supplemental testosterone won't make a difference. Other causes for loss of libido, such as side effects of some medications, anxiety or depression, painful sex, chronic illness, financial challenges, family dynamics (problems with children, sick parents), lack of privacy, mental illness, and marital strife must be considered.

How Long Will These Menopausal Symptoms Last?

"At 65, why am I still getting occasional hot flashes and regular night sweats?" Repeated studies have found that hot flashes sputter out for most women after 3 to 5 years in menopause, but some continue to have symptoms, generally not as severe, for 10 years or more. About one-third of women who take estrogen find that some of the symptoms of menopause return once they stop or as they taper off their treatment. Approximately 15 percent of women have hot flashes at ages 55 to 59, and 6.5 percent continue to have hot flashes up to age 65.[13]

Again, while we don't know the mechanism for hot flashes, night sweats, and some of the other symptoms of menopause, we know that low estrogen levels are the cause. The part of the brain that regulates temperature, the body's thermostat, isn't working properly. If you're experiencing hot flashes and night sweats, cutting out caffeine, alcohol, and spicy foods can help.

By the time many perimenopausal patients come to see me, they have already been to at least one other doctor, often an internist or a general practitioner. I find that many of the women seeking medical help for the early symptoms of perimenopause are put through a battery of costly tests and multiple doctor visits that come back negative. In an effort to help, doctors often prescribe antidepressants or sleeping pills for anxiety or sleeplessness, or get EKGs to see if there may be a heart problem, instead of determining that the symptoms are perimenopause related. If you are experiencing the symptoms described in this chapter, consider talking with your gynecologist or other health-care provider familiar with perimenopause and menopause.

Also know that even though your estrogen levels are dropping during perimenopause, you can still become pregnant. Unless you want

BARBARA had her last period at the age of 54. She finally decided to seek help because she suffered from hot flashes and night sweats that affected her quality of life. "My body was like the engine in a luxury sports car that goes from zero to 60 in a matter of seconds. It was as if someone was holding the accelerator to the floor and sweat suddenly began to pour out from everywhere at least 12 times a day. Every night my back became so hot, I thought someone would be able to fry an egg on it. Taking oral estrogen plus progesterone did the trick. At age 65, I've tried to stop taking it, but the symptoms came right back. I'm just not giving up my HT."

to get pregnant, be sure to use a reliable method of birth control until you have gone 12 months without a period. Many women choose to use a diaphragm, condoms, or an IUD in perimenopause. Every year or so one of my patients comes in with a "surprise" pregnancy. As Yogi Berra said, "It ain't over till it's over."

What Happens When I Stop Hormone Therapy?

Stopping HT is a big decision and can have many ramifications. As one study cited:

- If you had hot flashes before you started HT or you start taking hormones specifically for hot flashes, you are more likely to get them back. Smokers are also more likely to have hot flashes again.

- Hot flashes are likely to restart within a month of stopping HT. Keep a diary of your symptoms. More than half of women have no symptoms 3 years after stopping treatment and another third have only mild symptoms. Also, sleep difficulty, fatigue, moodiness, bladder issues, and joint pain may return. If symptoms do return, speak with your doctor. Download a free menopause symptoms diary at www.EstrogenFixBook.com /Menopause-Symptoms-Diary.

Women Who Should NOT Use Hormone Therapy

According to the FDA, do *not* take HT if you have a current or past history of any of the following:

- Breast or endometrial cancers
- Blood clots, particularly in the lungs, eyes, or deep veins
- Heart attack, stroke, or TIA (transient ischemic attack)
- Liver disease or liver problems
- Current pregnancy
- Undiagnosed uterine bleeding

While the study cited[15, 16] says that going "cold turkey" off estrogen does not seem to be better or worse than tapering off the medication, that hasn't been the experience of many of my patients. I do not advise going cold turkey for two reasons. First, I prefer tapering off the medication over a few months because it seems to work better in coming off the medication. There is a second reason I believe women should taper off their hormones, particularly if they are taking Prempro, and that has to do with a possible increased risk of heart attack from going cold turkey.[17] According to Dr. Phil Sarrel of Yale University, the effects of Premarin will wear off in about 2 weeks, but the effects of Provera can last for up to 12 weeks.[18] Thus, going cold turkey will cause an imbalance of the negative effects of Provera to dominate; the main negative effect is narrowing of the coronary arteries, which could precipitate a heart attack or stroke. This point was emphasized in a study of over 332,202 Finnish women who were followed for 15 years after they decided to discontinue their HT. Women less than 60 years who discontinued their HT had a 26 to 66 precent increased risk of death from heart attack and stroke within a year of stopping therapy than women who continued taking HT.[19] This underscores the importance of talking with your healthcare provider about how and when to discontinue HT. The reasons this happens has to do with the fact that estrogen promotes hormones in the blood vessels that dilate blood vessels and inhibits hormones that constrict them. We'll discuss this more in Chapter 5, The Estrogen Fix and Your Heart.

Chapter 3

Your Estrogen Fix: Choosing the Right Hormone Therapy for You

The estrogen window is a powerful concept that can transform your life for the better, and it is incredibly simple to understand. Once you do, you can begin taking advantage of your estrogen fix to reduce your anxiety about taking ET or EPT, lessen your potential risks of taking it, and have a much clearer and easier conversation with your health-care provider.

Why does the estrogen window matter for an estrogen fix? Just as your body has a biological clock with a reproductive window during which you can become pregnant, it also has an estrogen window, a time during which taking estrogen is most effective and the risks of taking it are the lowest they can be.

It's easy to know when your estrogen window opens; it's the moment you enter menopause. If you go into early or premature menopause in your twenties or thirties, your window opens then. In fact, women who go into early or premature menopause or surgical menopause[1, 2] derive even greater benefits from starting estrogen while their estrogen window is open because not doing so carries greater risks for sexual dysfunction, osteoporosis, heart disease, psychiatric disorders such as depression, anxiety, dementia,[3] and possibly suicide and breast cancer. If you enter menopause later in life, say at age 55, your estrogen window opens then.

Whether to take or use estrogen is an individual decision. If you are having moderate to severe menopausal symptoms and have a history of breast or endometrial cancer, blood clots, stroke, or severe heart disease, estrogen is likely not a good first choice for you. Estrogen alternatives are described on page 61 for women with medical histories that make it inadvisable to take estrogen. The estrogen window won't make estrogen safe for those women, though should they choose to take HT anyway, it will be the safest time to begin treatment.

The Estrogen Fix does not suggest that you must go on estrogen even if you have no medical reason to avoid it. I know there are women who for personal reasons don't want to take hormones. I respect their opinions, and for them there are estrogen alternatives. I also know that many of the women who avoid estrogen for personal reasons do so because they are afraid. The misinformation surrounding EPT and ET since the 2002 Women's Health Initiative (WHI) study and many others created such a phobia for estrogen that a generation of women suffered the symptoms and potential consequences of menopause; these fears were caused by a study that was inappropriately designed and analyzed. Premarin (or estrogen alone) and Prempro (or estrogen plus a progestogen) are two different stories, and their potential risks should be viewed differently. And neither of them can be fully understood without understanding the estrogen window.

In addition, the information in *The Estrogen Fix* does not have to apply to a woman who primarily wants to take estrogen vaginally to eliminate vaginal dryness, painful sex, or bladder symptoms, especially recurring bladder infections. If you are struggling with those symptoms, vaginal estrogen will be of enormous benefit. Vaginal estrogen can be used at any time in life, and you will have fewer symptoms with minimal risk. Your estrogen window for vaginal estrogen always remains open; it never closes. And though small amounts of estrogen may enter your bloodstream from the vaginal estrogen, the amounts are believed to be too small to cause medical problems. As you might expect, vaginal estrogen generally is not a treatment for hot flashes, prevention of osteoporosis, heart disease, or other major health problems; it is a treatment for the vaginal tissues and bladder—a condition now known as genitourinary syndrome (GSM) of menopause and formerly known as vulvovaginal atrophy (VVA). An exception is Femring, which contains high enough levels of estrogen to be absorbed and treat hot flashes.

Because vaginal estrogen is, of course, estrogen, the FDA requires that a "black box" warning be put on the package insert of all those products. That package insert states that taking estrogen can cause breast cancer and other findings of the 2002 WHI study. The impact of that black box warning has been to frighten most women away from using vaginal estrogen because they fear it will cause breast cancer. There is no evidence of any kind that this is true. In fact, in March, 2016, the American College of Obstetricians and Gynecologists published their committee opinion number 659 that stated that even women with estrogen-receptor positive breast cancer, either in the past or currently under treatment, could take vaginal estrogen if nonhormonal treatments failed, and that there was no evidence of an increased risk of cancer recurrence among women who do so.[4] How much estrogen actually gets into the bloodstream? According to psychologist and sex therapist Dr. Sheryl Kingsberg, if you used the vaginal estrogen Vagifem for an entire year, the amount of estrogen that would get into the bloodstream would be equivalent to taking one birth control pill.

There are doctors who may recommend that some women with moderate to severe symptoms during perimenopause take estrogen only, progesterone only, or a combination of both. If it makes sense to you and to your doctor to open your estrogen window a little bit earlier, that's okay. Starting estrogen as your own estrogen levels are fluctuating in a downward direction is a common treatment in perimenopause and helps prevent plaque from building up in your arteries, your vaginal and skin tissues from thinning, your bones from losing calcium, and hot flashes from fogging up your brain. All good.

If you have had your uterus removed (hysterectomy) and you need to take estrogen only, the story is really much simpler and more bulletproof. Women taking estrogen only (ET) from the time of menopause have lower risks of Alzheimer's disease, heart disease, and breast cancer. Realize I didn't say you can't or won't get any of these problems if you take ET. Life doesn't work that way. But you will be less likely to get those diseases by taking estrogen only than by not taking it.

Following is a table of oral estrogens available in the United States and Canada. As you can see, there are many types and brands. This table will help you understand their differences.

Oral Estrogen Therapy for Menopause

WHAT IT IS	NAME	DOSAGE IN MILLIGRAMS (MG)	USAGE
Conjugated estrogens—nonhuman natural estrogens that contain at least 10 estrogens from natural sources (urine of pregnant mares)	Premarin	0.3, 0.45, 0.625, 0.9, 1.25	Daily
Synthetic conjugated estrogens	Cenestin	0.3, 0.45, 0.625, 0.9, 1.25	Daily
	C.E.S.	0.3, 0.625, 0.9, 1.25	Daily
	PMS-Conjugated	0.3, 0.45, 0.625, 0.9, 1.25	Daily
	Enjuvia	0.3, 0.45, 0.625, 0.9, 1.25	Daily
Esterified estrogens	Menest	0.3, 0.625, 1.25, 2.5	Daily
	Estragyn	0.3, 0.625	Daily
17β-estradiol	Estrace, generics	0.5, 1.0, 2.0	Daily
Estropipate	Ogen	0.625, 1.25, 2.5	Daily
	Generics	0.625, 1.25, 5.0	Daily

North American Menopause Society, *Menopause Practice—A Clinician's Guide*, 5th Edition, 2014, p. 265.

What about women who have not had a hysterectomy and still have their uterus? In that situation, the estrogen window opens at the same time as for women who have had a hysterectomy, the moment they enter menopause. The details, however, differ from ET. The addition of progestogen to the estrogen (EPT) to protect the uterine lining from developing endometrial cancer carries slightly more potential risks than estrogen only. Even with that as a fact, the overwhelming information suggests that unless you have a medical reason not to take estrogen, the benefits outweigh the risks.[5]

Taking EPT in your estrogen window lowers the risk of osteoporosis-related fractures in women who are at risk of fractures before age 60. And while EPT may not lower the risk of heart disease and may not lower the risk of Alzheimer's disease unless the woman is in early menopause, it also doesn't increase the risk. So the benefits of taking the most effective treatment available for hot flashes during your estrogen window do not come with increased risk. There may be a slight risk of breast cancer with EPT, about the same risk of breast cancer as drinking one glass of wine daily and less risk than drinking two glasses daily.[6] However, a study of nearly half a million women found that for those who develop breast cancer after taking either ET or EPT, the chance of dying from their breast cancer was reduced by 50 percent.[7] The bar graph on the next page illustrates the relative risk of EPT and ET compared with other common conditions such as increased breast density, naturally occurring high levels of estrogen, and obesity leading to breast cancer. According to a global consensus on menopausal hormone therapy,[8] the risk of blood clots and strokes increases with oral EPT but is rare below age 60. The risk of blood clots is lower with transdermal estrogen than with oral estrogen[9] and highest if Provera is used.[10] If you do take estrogen, it is important to check with your doctor every 12 months, and if you develop any problems like bad headaches, blurred vision, or leg cramps, call your doctor to be sure you are not having a problem due to estrogen, progestogen, or other causes.

Estrogen-Progestogen Therapy for Menopause

WHAT IT IS	NAME	DOSAGE IN MILLIGRAMS (MG) OR MICROGRAMS (μG)	USAGE
Oral continuous cyclic regimen			
Conjugated estrogen (E) + medroxyprogesterone acetate (P)	Premphase	0.625 mg E + 5.0 mg P	(2 tablets: E days 1–14; E + P days 15–28)
Oral continuous combined regimen			
Conjugated estrogen (E) + medroxyprogesterone acetate (P)	Prempro	0.3 or 0.45 mg E + 1.5 mg P (1 tablet)	Daily
	Premplus	0.625 mg E + 2.5 or 5.0 mg P (1 tablet)	Daily
Ethinyl estradiol (E) + norethindrone acetate (P)	Femhrt	2.5 μg E + 0.5 mg P/tablet or 50 μg E + 1.0 mg P/tablet	Daily
17β-estradiol (E) + norethindrone acetate (P)	Activella	0.5 mg E + 0.1 mg P/tablet or 1 mg E + 0.5 mg P/tablet	Daily
17β-estradiol (E) + drospirenone (P)	Angeliq	0.5 mg E + 0.25 mg P/tablet, 1 mg E + 0.5 mg P/tablet, or 1 mg E + 1 mg P/tablet	Daily
Transdermal continuous combined regimen			
17β-estradiol (E) + norethindrone acetate (P)	Combi-Patch, Estalis	0.05 mg E + 0.14 mg P	9 cm² patch, twice/week
		0.05 mg E + 0.25 mg P	16 cm² patch, twice/week
17β-estradiol (E) + levonorgestrel (P)	Climara Pro	0.045 mg E + 0.015 mg P	22 cm² patch, once/week

North American Menopause Society, *Menopause Practice—A Clinician's Guide,* *5th Edition,* 2014, p. 268.

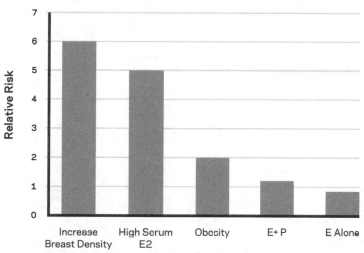

Challenges: Counseling Breast Cancer Risk and Hormone Therapy: Overall Perspective

A relative risk of 1 means no increased risk. Estrogen alone is a <1, meaning a reduced risk.

Premature or Early Menopause

Early menopause and premature menopause are special situations. I'm defining *early* menopause as occurring between the ages of 40 and 45; *premature* menopause occurs when a woman enters menopause before age 40. Either of these deprives a young woman of estrogen very early in her life and well before the average age of natural menopause. For that reason, a woman who experiences premature or early menopause will potentially live a much longer time without estrogen than the majority of women.

There is very clear evidence that in this group of women, not using estrogen increases their risk of sexual dysfunction, osteoporosis, heart disease, and psychiatric disorders such as depression, anxiety, and dementia.[11, 12] To lower the risk of dementia, it's best to take estrogen for at least 10 years.[13] In a review of the world literature, the most powerful of the four medications known to lower the risk of Alzheimer's disease is estrogen.[14] An important fact is that approximately 25 percent of women never fill their estrogen prescription, and many forget to take it or don't take it consistently.[15, 16] We also know that at the time of a hysterectomy, 40 percent of women are provided estrogen by their gynecologists, but when checked 10 months after, only 25 percent are using it. To get the most benefit, women in early or premature menopause (unless there is a

Estrogen Equivalent Dosages for Menopause

Oral	
Conjugated estrogen	0.625 mg
Synthetic conjugated estrogen	0.625 mg
Esterified estrogens—oral synthetic estrogen mixtures; example Menest—not for use for osteoporosis	0.625 mg
Estropipate (0.75 mg)	0.625 mg
Ethinyl estradiol	1.0 mg
Transdermal/topical	
Estradiol patch	0.05 mg–0.1 mg
Estradiol gel	1.5 mg/2 metered dosages
Vaginal	
Conjugated estrogens	0.3125 mg
17β-estradiol	0.5 mg

North American Menopause Society, *Menopause Practice—A Clinician's Guide*, 5th Edition, 2014, p. 268.

medical reason why they should not) should start ET or EPT at the time of menopause, or as soon afterward as possible, and continue taking it for at least until the average age of natural menopause, which is 51. Fifty-one, however, is the average age of menopause and the time when most women start ET or EPT. If a woman has been taking ET throughout her estrogen window, the benefits will continue without increased risk, at least for another decade. (We'll talk more about this in Chapter 6.) For EPT this information is still being analyzed, but extending the estrogen window use for another 5 years seems to make sense. About 43 percent of women[17, 18] at the time of menopause will have some form of sexual discomfort, but if their estrogen levels are low at a younger age and estrogen isn't replaced, by 7 years later that percentage will be 88 percent.[19, 20] This is just one more very important reason to be sure you are aware of your estrogen window so you can start taking estrogen.

What If You're Past Your Estrogen Window?

This question is still being answered as new data continue to be released. ET and EPT are considered medications that in general should not be given after age 60 because of the increased risk of dementia and heart disease and other problems. In many cases, doctors and health-care systems are being evaluated and scored on their care of patients, and giving HT to women over age 65 is considered a negative behavior because they are seen as giving a "potentially inappropriate medication" (PIM). Negative behaviors lower their scores and cause them to look like poor providers on Internet sites and other places that share such information. The PIM scores originated in 1991 when Mark H. Beers, a geriatrician, published a list of medications that seemed to affect older patients more negatively than younger patients.[21] His list was updated several more times, and when that happened in 2003 after the 2002 WHI, he included both oral and transdermal estrogen, with or without progestogens. Although the list was modified in 2012 to use estrogen with caution, more than 90 percent of health-care plans in the United States plus Medicare see estrogen for women over 65 as a red flag and will often deny its coverage. As you will discover, the estrogen window stays open much longer for ET, and for both ET and EPT, there is information that in certain situations, these medications can be given even longer. In fact, the latest position paper on the hormone therapy in menopause, released in October 2016, found no scientific evidence that women already taking estrogen cannot continue to take it if they have ongoing symptoms.[22] Beginning estrogen after the estrogen window closes, as mentioned above, is still being evaluated.

Almost half of postmenopausal women (42 percent) aged 60 to 65 still have at least some hot flashes, 6.5 percent still have moderate to severe hot flashes (see table on the next page), and nearly two-thirds report some sexual symptoms.[23] And symptoms don't end there for

Understanding Progestogens

Progestogens (sometimes spelled progestagens or gestagens) are a class of steroid hormones that act on the progesterone receptor (PR). The progestogen you likely know is progesterone (P4). The body also makes the progestogens in 17-hydroxyprogesterone, 5α-dihydroprogesterone, and 11-deoxycorticosterone. Synthetic progestogens are called progestins.[24] However, although technically not accurate, the terms *progesterone*, *progestogen*, and *progestin* are sometimes interchanged in both scientific literature and in clinical settings.

some women. For that reason the North American Menopause Society and the American College of Obstetricians and Gynecologists have issued statements that on an individualized basis, HT should be continued at the lowest effective dose if the perceived benefits outweigh the risks. So for now, it has to be realized that a large percentage of women will have significant symptoms that last longer than their estrogen window, and they are in a catch-22. Talk with your doctor about your potential risks versus benefits. Estrogen may still be right for you. Vaginal estrogen is something that almost every woman will still be able to consider. The North American Menopause Society has issued their recommendation for offering women estrogen after age 65 (see pages 58–59), and ACOG had published a committee report in March 2016 stating that even women diagnosed with estrogen receptor positive breast cancer can take vaginal estrogen if nonhormonal treatments are ineffective without worry of compromising cancer treatment or increasing the risk of recurrence. You can also consider alternatives to estrogen, and those can be taken together with vaginal estrogen.

Percentage of Women Experiencing Moderate to Severe Hot Flashes by Age

AGE GROUP	% HOT FLASHES
< 55	28.5
55–59	15.1
60–65	6.5

Which Hormone Therapy Regimen Is Right for You?

If you choose to take ET or EPT, you and your health-care provider have to decide which one of the four options that combine estrogen and progesterone is the right choice for you. One causes monthly bleeding, and two are intended to eliminate bleeding altogether. The fourth regimen is the newest and in theory may reduce the risk of breast cancer. These four regimens differ in the type of estrogen and progestogen used, and in the dosing pattern of the progestogen choice. The sequential, the continuous-combined, and the intermittent #1 regimens are all variations of standard EPT protocols. They all contain combinations of estrogen and progestogen for multiple days of each month. The intermittent #2 protocol limits the amount of progesterone in an attempt to reduce the potential risk of adding any progestogen. How long to take these types of regimens is discussed beginning on page 55.

Types of EPT Protocols

1. The sequential or continuous-cyclic regimen is designed to mimic a natural menstrual cycle. Estrogen is taken every day and a progestogen, preferably progesterone, is added for the last 10 to 14 days of each month. This hormone pattern is similar to what happens in a natural menstrual cycle because of its effect on the uterine lining. And as with women who have menstrual cycles, this regimen will frequently cause bleeding within days after the last progesterone dose that resembles a normal period, although it may be lighter. This method is similar to many birth control pills and prevents pregnancy as well as provides HT. You will not ovulate even though you are bleeding monthly.

2. The continuous-combined regimen employs a daily regimen of both estrogen and progesterone throughout the month. If your goal is to eliminate all bleeding, this is a good method to try. It keeps the uterine lining thin so that after a few months to 1 year of treatment, bleeding is greatly reduced or eliminated. Bleeding is more likely to stop if you are a few years into menopause rather than at the beginning.

3. The intermittent #1 regimen uses a lower total amount of progesterone and alternates 3 days of estrogen alone with 3 days of estrogen and progesterone. It is based on a theory that during the estrogen-only days, the uterine lining becomes more sensitized to progesterone. So adding progesterone for only a short time at a low dose can cause the uterine lining to become thin. Whether this method is comparable or superior to the continuous-combined regimen needs further study. At present, this regimen is not commonly used.

4. The intermittent #2 regimen came into use after an article appeared in the April 2012 issue of the *Journal of the American Medical Association* that found that women who take only estrogen without a progestin have a 23 percent lower risk of breast cancer. This is particularly good news for women who have had a hysterectomy and need only ET.

The Four Ways of Taking Estrogen and Progestogen

Sequential	Take estrogen every day. Take progestogen last 10–14 days per month.
Continuous-combined	Take estrogen every day. Take progestogen every day.
Intermittent number 1	Take estrogen every day. Take progestogen for 3 days; stop taking progestogen for 3 days.
Intermittent number 2	Take estrogen every day. Take progestogen for 10–14 days every 3–6 months.

The catch is that if a woman has her uterus and takes estrogen, she must also take progesterone to lower her risk of getting uterine cancer. To make sure that a woman with a uterus who takes estrogen has the lowest risk of both breast cancer and uterine cancer, she should take a progestogen for 12 days every 3 to 4 months, and possibly as occasionally as every 6 months. In these situations, I prescribe a bioidentical progesterone as the progestogen. To be on the safe side and to be certain there is no buildup of the uterine lining in women who have not had a hysterectomy, it's best to get a pelvic ultrasound every 1 to 2 years or to check the cells of the uterine lining with a simple office procedure called an endometrial biopsy. A new combined oral bioidentical estradiol and progesterone currently known as TX-001HR should soon to be available that significantly reduces hot flashes and causes virtually no abnormal buildup of the uterine lining.

How Much Estrogen Should You Take?

Because of the waxing and waning of your estrogen levels during perimenopause and menopause, symptoms such as hot flashes, night sweats, sleep deprivation, and others may be worse at certain times than others. They will come, go, and probably return. Those night sweats that sent you to the shower twice a night to cool off may have dissipated after 4 months, only to return another 4 months later, as your estrogen levels go up and down during this transitional time. Since this zigzagging, up-and-down hormone pattern is trending in a lower direction, over time your symptoms will lessen as your body adjusts to the lower estrogen levels.

My philosophy is that women should start with a low dose. The biggest impact on symptom relief is usually between prescribing some versus none. After about 1 to 3 months, if symptoms are not significantly improved, I increase the dosage up to the next level and repeat every month or two until my patient is comfortable. Most women only require one or two adjustments at most, and many will feel great at the lowest dosages. Start low; you can always add more.

Low-Dose Estrogen Options

Transdermal	14 µg/day, 37.5 µg/day
17β-estradiol	1 mg/day (oral)
Conjugated estrogen, esterified estrogen	0.3 mg, 0.45 mg (oral)

Progestogen Dose Required to Protect the Uterine Lining with Estrogen

	SEQUENTIAL EPT (PROGESTOGEN DAILY 10-14 D/MO)	CONTINUOUS-COMBINED EPT (DAILY)
Oral tablets		
Medroxyprogesterone acetate (MPA) (Provera)	5 mg	2.5 mg
Norethindrone	0.35 mg–0.7 mg	0.35 mg
Norethindrone acetate	2.5 mg	0.5 mg–1 mg
Micronized progesterone (bioidentical)	200 mg	100 mg
Intrauterine system		
Levonorgestrel*		20 µg/d or 6 µg/d
Mirena IUD*		20 µg/d or 6 µg/d
Vaginal		
Progesterone gel	45 mg	45 mg

North American Menopause Society, *Menopause Practice—A Clinician's Guide, 5th Edition*, 2014, p. 274.

*Not approved for this purpose

Estrogen Delivery Systems

There are a number of ways to take estrogen, and each one has its pluses and minuses, as you'll read below.

Tablets: Swallowing an estrogen-only or estrogen-progestogen tablet or pill is the most popular delivery system. Millions of women have taken a daily birth control pill, so taking HT by mouth seems familiar to them. Most women take them at bedtime. The estrogen pill Premarin has been studied more extensively than any other form of estrogen. HT tablets are absorbed from the intestines and pass through the liver and the enterohepatic circulation. Orally administered estrogen reduces LDL (bad) cholesterol levels and increases HDL (good) cholesterol levels in postmenopausal women with normal or elevated baseline lipid levels. Oral estrogen, particularly higher levels, is associated with an increased risk of blood clots. On the other hand, with a lower dose of conjugated estrogen of 0.45 milligrams or less and the estrogen estradiol, it's less likely that blood clots will develop.[25] Dosages are typically once daily, although estradiol tablets don't last as long in the bloodstream and may require twice-daily dosages. For symptoms of menopause, such as hot flashes, relief may come as soon as a few days or may take up to 4 to 6 weeks.

Equivalent Dosages of Different Estrogen Delivery Systems

Oral	
Conjugated estrogens	0.625 mg
Synthetic conjugated estrogens	0.625 mg
Esterified estrogens	0.625 mg
Estropipate (0.75 mg)	0.625 mg
Ethinyl estradiol	0.005 mg–0.015mg
17β-estradiol	1.0 mg
Transdermal/topical	
Estradiol patch	0.05 mg–0.1 mg
Estradiol gel	1.5 mg/2 metered doses
Vaginal	
Conjugated estrogens	0.3125 mg
17β-estradiol	0.5 mg

North American Menopause Society, *Menopause Practice—A Clinician's Guide*, *5th Edition*, 2014, p. 269.

Topical creams, gels, and sprays: These products contain estrogen that is applied directly to the skin. Since you're not swallowing the pill, the estrogen bypasses the liver, and that lessens the risks of stroke and blood clots.

On the other hand, some women have skin that can react negatively to estrogen or doesn't absorb creams, gels, or sprays well. These must be applied specifically as directed. First, thoroughly wash your hands before and after applying estrogen, so it doesn't come in contact with your partner or other people, especially children, or pets that may lick the skin area covered with estrogen. If someone else does come into direct contact with the product within the first 2 hours after applying it, have them immediately wash the specific area with soap and water. Covering your skin with clothing for a few hours where the product was applied decreases any potential risk of the cream, gel, or spray coming into contact with another partner, child, or pet. There are a number of reports of dogs licking the area where estrogen was applied and then showing behavioral changes or mimicking being in heat.[26] While the dosages are typically once or twice daily, the amount spread or sprayed on the skin may vary slightly with each application. Compounding pharmacies prepare hormone creams by mixing a known amount of hormones into a container of cream or gel and then stirring it up. These preparations are not FDA approved and sometimes the actual dosage you receive of a compounded cream or gel may vary because of the mixing of the hormone. Most of these are bioidentical estrogen. As with oral estrogen, relief may come as soon as a few days or may take up to 4 to 6 weeks. Warning: Applying sunscreen before applying a patch, cream, or gel may increase your exposure to estrogen. Applying sunscreen before applying a spray does not affect estrogen exposure.

Adhesive patches: Adhesive patches vary from the size of a dime to the size of a silver dollar. Wash and dry your hands before touching the patch. Most contain bioidentical estradiol. Clean the area where the patch will be applied using a cotton ball and alcohol. The adhesive side sticks to the skin and transfers the hormone to the body. This is called transdermal. Place the patch on one side of the lower abdomen or on the upper back near the shoulder. Patches are changed and discarded and a new one applied to the opposite side once or twice weekly depending on which patch you use. If the patch begins to peel off before it's time to change it, cover it with a bandage or medical tape. Or take it off and heat the patch with a hair dryer set to low to help it stick back on. Patch dosages are very regulated by the FDA and carry the same amount of HT as every other patch, so there is no guessing whether you're getting the right dosage.

While patches carry lower risk of blood clots than oral estrogen, some women have an allergy to the adhesive or skin that doesn't allow for optimum penetration and absorption. Patches that have a reservoir of estradiol such as Estraderm are more likely to be irritating to the skin. Newer patches such as Vivelle or others I've listed in the table below, which use a matrix delivery system, are unlikely to cause skin sensitivity. Some women lead active lives, which may cause the patch to come off. Patches protect against the same things that other forms of estrogen do, and relief comes within days or up to 4 to 6 weeks, as with other forms of estrogen.

Transdermal Estrogen Therapy for Menopause

WHAT IT IS	NAME	DOSAGE IN MILLIGRAMS (MG)	USAGE
17β-estradiol matrix patch	Alora	0.025, 0.05, 0.075, 0.1	Twice/week
	Climara	0.025, 0.0375, 0.05, 0.075, 0.1	Once/week
	Estradot	0.025, 0.0375, 0.05, 0.075, 0.1	Twice/week
	Menostar	0.014 (for osteoporosis only)	Once/week
	Minivelle	0.0375, 0.05, 0.075, 0.1	Twice/week
	Oesclim	0.025, 0.0375, 0.05, 0.075, 0.1	Twice/week
	Vivelle	0.025, 0.0375, 0.05, 0.075, 0.1	Twice/week
	Vivelle-Dot	0.025, 0.0375, 0.05, 0.075, 0.1	Once or twice/week
	Generics		
17β-estradiol reservoir patch	Estraderm	0.025, 0.05, 0.1	Twice/week
17β-estradiol gel	Divigel	0.025, 0.05, 0.1	Daily
	Elestrin	0.52	Daily
	EstroGel, Estrogel	0.75	Daily
17β-estradiol emulsion	Estrasorb	0.05	Daily (2 packets)
17β-estradiol spray	Evamist	0.021 mg/90 µL spray; to 1.5 mg/90 µL spray if needed	Daily

North American Menopause Society, *Menopause Practice—A Clinician's Guide,* *5th Edition,* 2014, p. 266.

Vaginal creams, suppositories, and tablets: Vaginal creams and suppositories with estrogen alone or an estrogen-progesterone (typically one or the other and not both, though compounded creams can contain both) combination are usually inserted with a plastic applicator. The directions that come with them are easy to follow. Vaginally applied estrogen tends to remain mostly in the vagina, but small amounts do enter the bloodstream. Vagifem estrogen tablets, which are inserted into the vagina, allow only modest amounts of estrogen to enter the bloodstream, but the dosage is quite low, so some women may not get adequate improvement of their vaginal dryness. Many women who are prescribed Vagifem on their own will double the dosage, which will slightly increase the amount that enters the bloodstream. That level will still be low, but oncologists who are asking their breast cancer patients not to take any estrogen may encourage not doing this. If you are in that situation, discuss it with your doctor or even get a second opinion; quality of life is also very important. A recent large study reported that women who take vaginal tablets are more likely to use them than women taking vaginal cream. The reasons offered were that the tablets were convenient and neat to apply.[27]

Vaginal Estrogen Therapy for Menopause

WHAT IT IS	NAME	DOSAGE IN GRAMS (G), MILLIGRAMS (MG), OR MICROGRAMS (μG)	USAGE
Vaginal creams			
17β-estradiol	Estrace	First 1–2 weeks: 2–4 g/d; then 1 g/1–3x/week (0.1 mg active ingredient/g)	Daily first 1–2 weeks then 1–3 times/week
Conjugated estrogen	Premarin	0.625 mg active ingredient/g	0.5–2 g/d for 21 days then off 7 days or twice/week
Estrone	Estragyn	2–4 g/d; 1 mg active ingredient/g	Dosage lowered once symptoms controlled
Vaginal rings			
17β-estradiol	Estring	The 2-mg ring releases 7.5 μg/d for 90 days	Change every 3 months for urogenital syndrome of menopause
Estradiol acetate	Femring	Rings contain 12.4 mg or 24.8 mg—release 0.05 mg/d or 0.10 mg/d estradiol for 90 days	For urogenital syndrome of menopause and hot flashes—levels in blood high enough to suggest adding progestogen
Vaginal tablet			
Estradiol hemi-hydrate	Vagifem	1 tablet daily x 2 weeks; then 1 tablet 2x/week; tablets contain 10 μg estradiol hemihydrate = 10 μg estradiol	For urogenital syndrome of menopause

North American Menopause Society, *Menopause Practice—A Clinician's Guide,* *5th Edition,* 2014, p. 267.

Pellets: Estrogen is also available as bioidentical pellets. They have been around a long time but are not as widely used as some of the other forms and are not FDA approved. Years ago, I went to London to visit the queen's gynecologist at that time, J. W. W. Studd, on Harley Street, to learn how to insert them; they were quite popular there. The line formed to receive them that Saturday morning went out the waiting room, down the steps, and around the corner. It comes in different dosages and is implanted under the skin with a small incision and an instrument about the width of a pencil. The small incision is closed with a stitch or an adhesive, and the stitch is removed in a day or two. The procedure is done with local anesthesia, and usually the pellets last for 4 to 6 months. They come in dosages of 25mg, 50mg, and 75mg. If you do use them, I recommend you have blood levels of estradiol drawn periodically as blood levels can be higher than the body naturally makes and can stay elevated for many months. I prefer FDA-approved delivery systems.

Vaginal ring: Vaginal rings deliver an estrogen dosage that enters the bloodstream. Though the dosage may be too small to guarantee protection against osteoporosis, it may help other symptoms, such as hot flashes and night sweats. Femring provides much higher blood levels than the Estring. To insert a vaginal ring, thoroughly wash and dry your hands before and after. It's like putting in a diaphragm. If you've never done that, ask your health-care provider to show you how to insert it. Choose a position that's comfortable for you, such as lying down, squatting, or standing with one leg propped up on a chair. Hold the ring between your thumb and index finger and press the opposite sides together. Gently push the folded ring as deeply as possible into the upper one-third of the vagina. If you have any discomfort, the ring is probably not inserted far enough into your vagina. Use your finger to gently push the ring farther into your vagina.

Your cervix will block the ring from going past the top of the vagina. If you've had a hysterectomy, just insert it gently in as far as you can. Either way, you can only insert it as far as the end of the vagina. If you feel the ring move during a bowel movement or when coughing, wash your hands and use a finger to push it back into place. If the ring is removed or falls out of the vagina for any reason, just rinse the ring with lukewarm water and reinsert it. A ring is usually left in place for 90 days, then replaced with a new one, so be sure to follow the dosing schedule carefully. Vaginal symptoms often improve within days, although it may take several weeks.

What Does Bioidentical Mean?

If you're confused by the term *bioidentical*, you are not alone. The term is often misused and misunderstood, so let's set the record straight. *Bioidentical* is not a scientific term. A bioidentical hormone simply means that its chemical structure is identical to the chemical structure of the hormone molecules produced in the human body. They are not natural, requiring 15 chemical reactions in a laboratory to produce them.[28] The bioidentical prescription estrogens are estrone, estradiol, and estriol. The most common bioidentical estrogen is estradiol.

The confusion sets in because many people believe that bioidentical hormones are safer and more natural than nonbioidentical hormones and can only be found in compounding pharmacies. Let's address each of these misunderstandings.

1. Bioidentical hormones per se are neither safer nor riskier than non-bioidentical hormones. The risks and benefits of estrogen are similar whether the hormone is bioidentical or not. Bioidentical hormones have some specific benefits, such as the ability to measure bioidentical blood hormone levels in a blood test.

2. *Bioidentical* has become equated with the term *natural hormone therapy*, suggesting that bioidentical hormones exist naturally in plants in their final bioidentical form. In fact, "natural" can apply to any product where the principal ingredient comes from animals, plants, or minerals. Based on those criteria, because Premarin comes from the urine of pregnant mares, one could argue that Premarin is natural. The principal substances used to manufacture bioidentical estrogens do come from plants such as soybeans or wild yams, but the plant substances are estrogen precursors that must be chemically altered to create the final bioidentical chemical structure of estradiol. Our bodies don't have the ability to convert those precursors into the final product.

3. Bioidentical hormones do not only come from a compounding pharmacy. Whether a bioidentical estradiol in the form of a patch, spray, vaginal ring, or cream is purchased from the pharmacist's shelf at a chain drugstore *or* mixed specifically for you at a compounding pharmacy, the bioidentical hormone will be exactly the same. Both chain drugstores and compounding pharmacies provide estrogens

that are produced from the same botanical plant sources. And whether you buy a bioidentical estrogen from a chain drugstore or a compounding pharmacy, it comes from the same plant source—the chemical plant.

The benefits of purchasing a bioidentical estrogen from a chain drugstore are that it is very tightly FDA regulated and has very rigorous quality controls.[29] Every prescription you fill will contain exactly what your doctor prescribed and exactly what is written on the packaging label. Every tablet in your prescription will contain precisely the same amount of hormone therapy as the other tablets. Each patch in your prescription will contain the same amount of hormone therapy as the other patches. Every delivery system will contain the same amount of estrogen or estrogen and progesterone as the other tablets, patches, rings, or creams.

The benefits of purchasing a bioidentical estrogen from a compounding pharmacy is that they can prepare—or compound—hormone therapy to any strength or dosage that is prescribed by your doctor. Compounding pharmacies can also provide hormones that are not currently available from chain drugstores or other FDA-approved drugstores. An example would be testosterone in dosages appropriate for women. The compounded prescription can also contain more than one hormone, which can be advantageous. This benefit is also a potential risk. Because compounded prescriptions are prepared uniquely and hand mixed, estrogen concentrations in any particular prescription may vary in dose from what your doctor ordered. Each estrogen batch may also vary slightly from one prescription to the next. As you will read below, this happens often.

Here's another way to explain compounded bioidentical hormones: Have you ever gone into an ice cream store and asked that M&M'S or another candy be mixed into your vanilla ice cream? While the server does his best to make sure that the candy is evenly distributed throughout the ice cream, one bite of ice cream may be packed with a dozen bits of candy, while the next one has none. Like your ice cream, a compounded cream, gel, or other medication from a compounding pharmacy may not be thoroughly and evenly mixed. The extent can vary from pharmacy to pharmacy or vendor to vendor or prescription to prescription.

Bioidentical hormones purchased at compounding pharmacies and as mentioned previously, in pellets, are not FDA approved. Compounding pharmacies were not even FDA regulated until after a November 2013[30] incident, when a compounding center shipped a contaminated anti-inflammatory that killed 63 people. *More* magazine and the Fund for Investigative Journalism commissioned lab tests of bioidentical hormones produced by 12 unregulated compounding pharmacies nationwide. The study found that women who use compounded bioidentical hormone therapy (BHT) were risking their health. Flora Research Laboratories evaluated 12 prescriptions gathered from 12 compounding companies in the United States. Flora's analysis revealed that these hormones were of unreliable potency and didn't meet the FDA's requirements for commercially manufactured drugs. "Doses in the pills tested fluctuated in a way that could increase the risk of uterine cancer because of a shortfall of the hormone progesterone." By that I mean that Flora found that the compounded prescriptions of estrogen tended to have much higher dosages than what was ordered, and the compounded prescriptions of progesterone tended to have much lower levels of progesterone than what was ordered. According to a survey on bioidentical hormones presented at the 2015 NAMS Annual Meeting, presented by Dr. Margery Gass, a small but steady number of women have developed endometrial cancer (of the uterine lining) while using compounded hormone therapy, even if they were taking compounded progesterone.[31] There were no reported cases of this happening from FDA-approved sources of EPT.

Most women don't realize compounded products are not FDA-approved. According to a survey published in 2015 by NAMS, when asked, "Do you believe that bio-identical hormone therapies compounded at a specialty pharmacy are FDA-approved?" only 14 percent of women correctly answered "no." The majority—76 percent—weren't sure and 10 percent incorrectly answered "yes."[32]

A 2016 Scientific Statement by the Endocrine Society took a strong stance against compounded bioidentical hormone therapy. Their report clarified that there is no scientific evidence to support that compounded hormone therapy is more effective or less likely to cause cancer.[33] The report also points out that the compounding pharmacies are not required to include a "black box" warning that all FDA-approved estrogen products are required to provide stating estrogen's potential risks, and there are no large, long-term, randomized, double-blind, placebo-controlled studies that have determined the effectiveness, safety, or adverse effects of custom-compounded bioidentical hormones. There is also no scientific evidence that a correlation exists between a patient's symptoms and salivary hormones.

In presentations at the 2015 NAMS Annual Meeting by Drs. Wulf Utian and Margery Gass, the common finding of too much estrogen and not enough progesterone from filled compounded prescriptions was emphasized as a health risk.

How did compounded hormones become so popular? When the negative results of the WHI study were first published in 2002, women suddenly stopped taking estrogen, yet they were clamoring for something to relieve the symptoms of menopause. Suzanne Somers and other celebrities touted bioidentical hormones as safer to use, and women were desperate to find "safer" estrogen. Many doctors were not eager to prescribe conjugated estrogens like the ones in the WHI study. The concept took off.

According to the same 2015 NAMS presentations, among women who have ever used hormone therapy, many used compounded hormone therapy (C-HT) (see table below). The main reasons they gave for using it were that they believed it was safer and had other nonproven benefits.

Percentage of Women by Age Who Have Used Compounded Hormone Therapy

AGES 40-49	50-64	65-74	75-84
41	32	25	15

The bottom line: While there are many excellent compounding pharmacies, and compounding pharmacies are increasing their internal regulation to ensure customers get what their doctors order, industry regulations are not yet comparable to those of pharmaceutical companies. There is no scientific proof that custom-compounded bioidentical hormone therapy is any safer or more effective than FDA-approved bioidentical hormone therapies. My advice is that if you are taking compounded hormone therapy, be certain your health-care provider checks your uterine lining. Before thinking that compounded hormone therapy is safer or the only way to get the dosage you need, realize that both FDA-approved bioidentical estrogen and progesterone are available in multiple dosages and forms from drugstores and chain stores and will contain the dose that was ordered; and their safety, risks, and benefits will have been studied.

When Does Your Estrogen Window Close?

This is a question whose answer is still being refined. For that reason, it will require ongoing discussions with your doctor at your annual exams. I always tell my patients that ET and EPT is a 5-year renewable option for two reasons: (1) In 5 years new information may change recommendations, and (2) in 5 years you may change.

In general, the estrogen window is a decade-long time frame between the ages of 50 and 60, or 10 years from the time of menopause. And in general it is true. To make it a little more specific, here are my recommendations for the estrogen window based on my findings. Where appropriate, I've also added in the most recent consensus of the menopause experts throughout the world.

Women taking ET: Women who have had a hysterectomy with no medical reason not to take estrogen have the most complete information about taking estrogen and the details of their estrogen window.

If you are a woman with *low risk* of cardiovascular heart disease based on a predictive risk score that considers whether or not you smoke or have diabetes, and that considers your blood pressure and blood cholesterol panel, you can take ET for 5 years from the onset of menopause[34] and, together with your doctor, extend your estrogen window for an additional 5 years for a total of 10 years. Newer information based on nearly 500,000 women suggests that the window for taking estrogen only (ET) may possibly be open for an additional 5 years or more.[35] In fact, women who stopped estrogen earlier had more coronary heart disease and stroke and died earlier than those who continued to take it for longer periods of time. To assess your 10-year risk of cardiovascular heart disease, visit imedicalapps.com/2014/04/ascvd-risk-estimator-app/.

If you have *moderate risk* of cardiovascular heart disease, you can still take ET for 10 years from the moment of menopause, but transdermal estrogen rather than oral may be safer because it is associated with lower risk of blood clots.

If you are at *high risk* of cardiovascular heart disease at the time of beginning ET, it's best not to choose ET. Consider an alternative to ET first. But here is the good news: If you were at low risk at the time you began ET and started it well within your estrogen window, close to the beginning of menopause, and continued to take it throughout the 10 years that followed, you may be able to continue ET for another 7 years. I'm basing this information on the 2004 WHI study,[36, 37] which was done in women aged 50 to 79. While there was a slightly increased risk of stroke, there was no increased risk of heart disease or breast cancer and a reduction in the risk of hip fracture. The large study of nearly 500,000 women I mentioned previously also found that staying on estrogen (in the case of that study, estradiol) also lowered the risk of stroke. So if you are taking ET and began it during your estrogen window, the evidence is suggesting your window stays open even beyond the 10 years since menopause. This of course will depend on your seeing your doctor annually to make sure no new risk factors develop.

Women taking EPT: Women who have their uterus must take a combination of estrogen and some form of a progestogen to protect the lining.[38] I believe women at low to moderate risk of cardiovascular heart disease or who do not have other medical reasons not to take EPT can take EPT for up to 5 years with at most minimal risk if they begin taking it within their estrogen window along with annual exams by their doctor. As I mentioned earlier, estrogen is a 5-year renewable option, and depending on the individual, treatment may be continued or discontinued at that time. Either way, it's an opportunity to gain a window of valuable benefits and symptom relief from EPT. The large Finnish study of nearly 500,000 women found that taking EPT for 10 years also lowered the risk of death from heart disease for women taking estradiol plus some type of progestogen.[39] So the 10-year window seems a safe interval for most women who start within their estrogen window. It may be that their population had a safer outcome than what was reported in the WHI because the women in Finland all use oral or transdermal estradiol, not conjugated estrogen, and most of the progestogen ordered was a synthetic progestin called norethisterone acetate and not Provera.

Most of the worrisome results reported in the WHI studies were in women using a combination of Premarin and medroxyprogesterone acetate (Provera). The ET-only arm of the study, using Premarin only, had many fewer bad outcomes. I, and many other doctors, believed that the greater risk was due to Provera,[40] not Premarin. Provera has some non-progesterone effects that include enhancing the potency of estrogen and narrowing blood vessels.[41] For that reason, I rarely prescribe Provera as the progestin to take with estrogen. How can this change the way doctors treat women who still have their uterus? Here are four options that can be used with fewer risks than EPT. I use them, and you can discuss them with your doctor as alternative approaches.

Alternative Regimens for EPT

1. **Transdermal patch:** We've already discussed how the transdermal approach has lower risk of blood clots. Bioidentical creams, gels, or pellets can also be used for the same reasons, though they are much less studied. Taking oral conjugated estrogen at dosages of ≤ 0.45 milligram or estradiol at dosages of ≤ 1 milligram may also lower the risk of blood clots.

2. **Bioidentical progesterone:** Bioidentical (see page 51, "What Does Bioidentical Mean?") progesterone appears to have less risk of breast cancer in postmenopausal women.[42, 43] Remember, ET does not increase the risk of breast cancer, and if taken early in your estrogen window, lowers breast cancer risk. In addition to using the bioidentical progesterone each month, treating a woman's lining with progesterone every 3 to 4 months or even every 6 months[44] limits the amount of progesterone the woman is exposed to but is often enough to protect her uterine lining from developing cancer. With these intermittent regimens, it's important to have an annual ultrasound or endometrial biopsy to be certain that no endometrial hyperplasia (increased cell production) of the uterine lining occurs.

3. **Progesterone-secreting IUD (intrauterine device):** It may seem odd to suggest a form of birth control in menopause, but sometimes that's what I do. The Mirena IUD contains the synthetic progestin levonorgestrel, which releases the progestin over a 5-year period of time. While this IUD is not marketed for this purpose, the progestin within it does help protect the lining of the uterus from the effects of estrogen. Very low levels of the progestin get into the bloodstream, but the main impact of combining Mirena with an estrogen virtually eliminates progesterone and allows the estrogen to work almost like ET. See page 77 on estrogen and breast cancer risk in women who have the BRCA or breast cancer gene.

4. **Duavee:** The FDA approved Duavee on October 3, 2013, for treatment of moderate-to-severe hot flashes and for prevention of osteoporosis. The medication contains a combination of Premarin and

HT: Major Points of Agreement

The North American Menopause Society, the American Society for Reproductive Medicine, and the Endocrine Society take the position that most healthy, recently menopausal women can use hormone therapy for relief of their symptoms of hot flashes and vaginal dryness if they choose to do so. These medical organizations also agree that women should know the facts about hormone therapy. Below are the major points of agreement among these societies.

- Hormone therapy reduces menopausal symptoms.

- Hormone therapy is the most effective treatment for menopausal symptoms such as hot flashes and vaginal dryness. If women have only vaginal dryness or discomfort with intercourse, the preferred treatments are low doses of vaginal estrogen.

- Hot flashes generally require an adequate dose of estrogen therapy that will have an effect on the entire body. Women who still have a uterus need to take a progestogen (progesterone or a similar product) along with the estrogen to prevent cancer of the uterus. Five years or less is usually the recommended dura-

bazedoxifene,[45] a selective estrogen receptor modulator (SERM) that is protective of bone health and of the uterine lining, and may be protective for breast tissue from developing breast cancer. This allows women who are worried about breast-associated risks from taking estrogen to take it with what appears to be greater safety. Duavee causes less breast tenderness than Prempro and does not increase breast density, which makes mammograms easier to read (see Chapter 4).[46] It has also been found to improve vaginal dryness, improve sleep, and not increase vaginal bleeding.[47] Symptom relief is typically within 3 to 6 weeks and improvement in the bone density is seen by 6 months. The medication has not been studied in women with breast cancer. Because it contains an estrogen, the medication's safety warnings contain the same warnings that are present on all estrogen products.

tion of use for this combined treatment, but the length of time can be individualized for each woman and is often extended.

- Women who have had their uterus removed can take estrogen alone. Because of the apparent greater safety of estrogen alone, there may be more flexibility in how long these women can safely use estrogen therapy.

Hormone Therapy Risks

- Both estrogen therapy and estrogen with progestogen therapy increase the risk of blood clots in the legs and lungs, similar to birth control pills, patches, and rings. Although the risks of blood clots and strokes increase with either type of hormone therapy, the risk is rare in the 50-to-59 age group.

- A small increased risk of breast cancer is seen with 5 or more years of continuous estrogen-progestogen therapy, possibly earlier. The risk decreases after hormone therapy is stopped. Use of estrogen alone for an average of 7 years in the WHI trial did not increase the risk of breast cancer.[48]

Alternative Therapies: Non-Estrogen Approaches to the Symptoms of Menopause

Choices for the treatment of menopause and its symptoms are neither new nor limited to estrogen. In fact, if you look back to the 1899 *Merck's Manual,* recommendations included ammonia, camphor, cannabis indica (that's right, marijuana), eucalyptus, hot springs, opium, and suc ovarian (the "juice" from cow ovaries crushed up at the slaughterhouse). Interestingly, the cows' ovaries likely included some form of estrogen. More than a century later, some of the alternative approaches, such as herbs and supplements, mentioned on page 61 for dealing with menopause symptoms are so widely used that I often wonder why *they* are called alternative. In fact, the more accurate term is complementary.

Some women who come to see me about their menopausal symptoms prefer to try an herbal or botanical remedy or nutritional supplements. I never discourage them. I do tell them that with all remedies, "Everything works for some women, but nothing works for everyone." Perhaps your friend found that taking black cohosh, a plant native to North America, successfully diminished the intensity of her hot flashes, but you saw no relief after taking the same supplement. That's not surprising for at least two reasons: Different people have different experiences, and as you transition into and through menopause, your estrogen levels are also transitioning up and down, so sometimes things work for a while and then stop working. Here are some tips for taking over-the-counter remedies:

Set your expectations. While some alternative remedies may make some of your menopausal symptoms tolerable for a while, they don't have the potency of pharmaceuticals to make hot flashes and night sweats completely disappear like estrogen-based medications do. Hot flashes can be both intense and frequent. With alternative remedies, the best you can typically hope for is to lower the intensity and frequency of your hot flashes and night sweats. You may find that taking evening primrose oil or black cohosh modestly decreases the number of hot flashes you have from 12 to 10 a day, or that you wake up fewer times during the night because of hot flashes. If that's enough for you, then that's great.

Be patient. These remedies take time to build up in the body, so they have to be taken regularly, perhaps twice a day, for up to 2 to 3 months until results are noticeable. They also have a short half-life, the amount of time necessary for the dosage to be reduced to precisely one-half of a given concentration or amount. As a result, the effects of most over-the-counter remedies don't last more than about 12 hours. For more sustained levels, take it in two dosages, 12 hours apart.

Try one at a time. If you take three remedies at the same time and you see results in a few months' time, you won't know which one is helping, so give each one a chance for a few months to see if it works. That way you'll know what is and isn't working, and you won't have to buy and take two or three OTCs at a time.

Take it regularly. If you're going to take a supplement just once a day, take it at bedtime, so the potential benefits are released into your bloodstream when you are trying to sleep and help you at night with hot flashes and night sweats.

Realize the limitations. Alternative therapies do not provide the powerful, life-enhancing, ongoing benefits of ET or EPT. Whereas estrogen has been proven to have positive effects on heart, brain, and bone health, over-the-counter remedies have none or at best very few.

Popular Alternative Therapies for Symptoms of Menopause

Herbs and Plant-Based Therapies

Black cohosh. This substance, which is derived from a plant, is one of the first alternative remedies that women use to try to relieve the symptoms of menopause. It comes in 20-milligram tablets that should be divided and taken twice a day, preferably 12 hours apart. Remifemin is the one proprietary version on the market, but generic black cohosh tablets are available in pharmacies and health food stores and may be combined with other remedies in various manufacturers' proprietary blends. The North American Menopause Society reports black cohosh may be helpful in the very short term (6 months or less) for treatment of hot flashes, night sweats, and vaginal dryness, but not enough studies have been done to measure its effectiveness. Too much black cohosh can cause dizziness, nausea, severe headaches, stiffness, and trembling limbs. Occasional stomach pains and intestinal discomfort may also happen, and a slower pulse and perspiration have also been reported. Black cohosh may make your symptoms tolerable rather than intolerable and doesn't offer the other benefits to your bones, heart, and brain as seen with HT.

Chasteberry. Chasteberry, the dried, ripe fruit of the chaste tree (*Vitex agnus-castus*), has been used since antiquity and is mentioned in the early works of Hippocrates, Dioscorides, and Theophrastus. Hippocrates recommended the plant for injuries, inflammation, and swelling of the spleen and suggested using the leaves in wine to help control hemorrhages and the "passing of afterbirth." The name *agnus castus* comes from the Latin meaning "chaste lamb," because it was believed that its seeds taken as a drink had the ability to reduce sexual desire. The English name of chaste tree comes from the belief that taking the plant would suppress the libido of women. This, in turn, led to the practice of novice monks chewing the tree's leaves to suppress their libido.

Chasteberry is used in the United Kingdom to reduce hot flashes, much like black cohosh is favored in North America. Pour 1 cup of boiling water over 1 teaspoon of fresh berries and steep for 10 minutes to make tea.[49] Drink the tea up to three times daily. Or you can mix 1 milliliter of chasteberry tincture or extract into 1 cup of water three times a day. Occasional itching and welts have been reported, so stop if these symptoms occur.

Dong quai. Dong quai (*Angelica sinensis*) is a traditional Chinese herb that has become popular in North America as treatment for a variety of women's health concerns, among them menopausal symptoms. In China, dong quai is typically prescribed as part of a mixture that includes several other herbs in combination, but here it is typically sold as a single herb. Some menopausal women do report that dong quai helps relieve hot flashes, but there is little scientific evidence. In one study of 71 postmenopausal women, dong quai at a dose of 4.5 milligrams daily and a placebo were compared for their ability to reduce the number of hot flashes over a 24-week period of time.[50] According to this study, there were no differences in the number of hot flashes, thickness of the vagina, or a number of other symptoms including joint pain, insomnia, headaches, or fatigue between the two groups. If you want to try it, brew a tea by placing 1 teaspoon of the dried root in 1 cup of water, bringing it to a boil, and then simmering gently for 10 minutes. You can also use 1 milliliter of the tincture form of the herb three times daily. It may take several weeks to notice any relief in your hot flashes. Be aware that dong quai is a mild laxative and in some women may cause uterine cramps. A rash may also occur if you get too much sun while taking dong quai.

Estroven. Black cohosh, soy isoflavones, ginkgo biloba, melatonin, and other ingredients make up this over-the-counter supplement. Estroven comes in several formulas that are said to provide multisymptom relief. It is popular among my patients.

Evening primrose oil. The oil of evening primrose (*Oenothera biennis*) plant is one of the most frequently suggested alternative treatments for menopausal symptoms. It is native to North America, and I often see it growing wild along the roads in New England, especially along sandy beaches and the edges of woods. Native Americans consumed the leaves, roots, and seedpods for food and as prepared extracts for a variety of conditions. Today evening primrose is used for a number of different conditions including rheumatoid arthritis, eczema, multiple sclerosis, premenstrual syndrome (PMS), cardiovascular disorders, chronic fatigue syndrome, Raynaud's phenomenon, weight loss, endometriosis, and diabetes. Although a number of positive scientific studies suggest evening primrose oil for eczema and the other conditions mentioned above, I could find only one study on evening primrose relieving symptoms of menopause and, unfortunately, it showed no benefit over placebos for hot flashes.[51] That doesn't mean you shouldn't give it a try if nothing else is working. Evening primrose oil is usually well tolerated, although mild upset stomach, indigestion, nausea, softening of stools, and headache can occur. The recommended daily dosage of evening primrose oil is four 500-milligram capsules over the course of the day. I've had many patients try vitamin E or evening primrose oil tablets for hot flashes, but only rarely have had someone report that it's helped.

Flaxseeds. Flaxseeds are a rich source of protein, omega-3 fatty acids, calcium, potassium, B vitamins, and soluble fiber. They have been effective in reducing the intensity and frequency of hot flashes and night sweats in women, some who halved their hot flashes by stirring 2 tablespoons of ground flaxseeds (also called flax meal) into cereal, juice, or yogurt twice daily. Purchase ground flaxseeds (whole flaxseeds are indigestible) at supermarkets and health food stores, and refrigerate them once open so they don't go rancid. You can also buy flaxseed oil in the refrigerator sections of health food stores. Purchase flaxseed oil in opaque bottles, check the expiration date, and refrigerate at home. The oil should have a fresh, nutty aroma. If it smells like motor oil, it has turned rancid, and like any oil, should be discarded. You may see some benefits in 4 to 6 weeks.

I-cool. I-cool is a proprietary isoflavone enriched with vitamin D and calcium that is taken once daily to decrease the frequency and intensity of hot flashes and night sweats. The isoflavone's name is geniVida. It is a synthetic compound and appears to not cause allergies in people allergic to soy. I-cool is available in tablets or chewables and is a popular supplement.

Red clover. Red clover (*Trifolium pratense*), a plant that contains phytoestrogens or plant estrogens, has also been used for treatment of menopausal symptoms. Two clinical trials from Australia were unable to demonstrate that red clover extract was any better than using a placebo. However, another study found that a daily tablet of 40 milligrams of red clover did significantly reduce hot flashes.[52] There is still too little information to know whether or not red clover has any effect on the uterine lining or on breast tissue.[53] Also, because red clover contains coumarins, which have the ability to thin the blood, high dosages may cause this problem as well.

Take a 40-milligram supplement daily. Or brew 1 to 3 teaspoons of red clover tea in a cup of boiling water for 10 minutes three times a day. You can also dissolve 1 to 2 milliliters of red clover tincture in a glass of water and drink it three times a day. Allergic reactions may include itching and hives.

Soy. I think soy is a great source of phytoestrogens that works well for many women, particularly when symptoms are mild to moderate. So much so that at the time of the 2002 WHI report I wrote an entire book on the subject called *The Soy Solution for Menopause* that explained in detail its benefits and how to take it along with other complementary options. Soybeans are high in isoflavones, which are types of phytoestrogens, especially genistein and daidzein. Soy isoflavones, not soy protein, have been shown to be most beneficial for symptoms of menopause, but again, they don't offer the other benefits of ET and EPT. Soy can be taken in two ways: first, as a supplement of 50 or 100 milligrams twice a day— once in the morning, then again 12 hours later. The second option is to eat foods rich in soy, like soybeans, tofu, soy yogurt, soy nutrition bars, and soy milk. If you do go the food route, try to eat 25 to 40 grams of soy a day. Soy foods are also rich in calcium and good for lowering cholesterol. To be effective, add soy milk to herbal teas, decaffeinated coffee, or whole grain cereal in the morning; eat a handful of steamed edamame during the day; and dine on tofu at your evening meal. In other words, spread your soy consumption throughout the day for potential benefits.

In one study 40 percent of the women who ate soy showed a decrease in hot flashes and night sweats, while 30 percent of the women who took a soy placebo also showed a decrease in the same symptoms. Note: The difference was only 10 percent! Although not everyone agrees, I believe eating soy foods regularly can lower the frequency and intensity of hot flashes by as much as 30 to 50 percent, especially if the hot flashes are not severe. That may be just enough to make a huge difference in the quality of your day and your sleep. Some soy foods are a good source of protein and essential amino acids that have positive effects on bone and muscle health, and for maintaining blood pressure.

One very interesting study connects soy to the estrogen window.[54] In this study, which was a review of 10 placebo-controlled studies of soy to determine whether it improved cognition, the researchers found that soy isoflavones had a positive effect on improving cognition and visual memory in postmenopausal women and that it was most effective in women who began taking it before age 60. So it seems that the plant estrogen soy, like estrogen, has an estrogen window. Similar findings have been shown for soy for managment of depression.[55]

Because soy is a plant estrogen, there has been some concern that eating it may be harmful to breast cancer patients, since eating soy did encourage breast cancer in mice studies. Oncologists began recommending that their breast cancer patients avoid soy. With researchers talking about both potential benefits and harm, it is no wonder soy became and is still is a very confusing and controversial food.

Fortunately, within the past several years, research has cleared up much of the confusion on the relationship between soy and breast cancer. In an interview with me for *The Hot Years-My Menopause Magazine*, Dr. Mark Messina, one of the world's leading experts on soy, shared that in 2012, both the American Institute for Cancer Research and the American Cancer Society concluded that breast cancer patients could safely consume soy foods.[56] And in May 2013, after a comprehensive study published in the journal *Oncology*,[57] many renowned researchers reached a similar conclusion. It turns out that soybeans contain a number of compounds called *chemopreventives* that have the ability to inhibit, delay, or reverse cancer. Based on this new data, it appears that soy can be eaten or taken for the prevention of menopausal symptoms, even in breast cancer patients. In fact, in one survey, breast cancer survivors are six times as likely to report use of dietary soy than the general population.

Vitamins

Vitamin D$_3$. Most people associate vitamin D with bone health. Women, especially where I practice in the Northeast, often have low levels of vitamin D due to lack of exposure to sunshine. However, vitamin D levels seem to be low across the nation, even in many sunny areas. Vitamin D is essential for bone, heart, and muscle wellness and the absorption of calcium. Some of the women I treat have extremely low levels of vitamin D. I have found that some of the women who began taking vitamin D$_3$ to raise their levels to normal have seen their hot flashes reduced or, rarely, even eliminated. I'm not recommending vitamin D for treatment, but lowering hot flashes may be a very welcome by-product of bringing levels back to normal. Once levels do return to normal, it's important to stay on vitamin D supplements or low levels typically return.

Vitamin E. Vitamin E plays an important role in many neurological and other body functions. For the present time, the value of vitamin E for hot flashes seems minimal in studies, but, as I've said, even minimal relief from hot flashes and night sweats can be of value. If you do want to try it, take up to 1,000 IU daily. Check with your health-care provider if you are also taking aspirin or ginkgo biloba before adding vitamin E, as this combination may cause blood thinning that leads to easy bruising or, rarely, internal bleeding.

Vaginal Moisturizers

For women struggling with vaginal dryness, several vaginal moisturizers are available over the counter. Moisturizers are different than lubricants because they keep the vagina moist for more than just a few minutes after application. The most studied brand is Replens, which is applied daily with an applicator for approximately 1 week and then two to three times weekly. In a study conducted by Dr. Lila Nachtigall,[59] Replens given three times per week was compared with 2 grams daily of vaginal Premarin for a period of 12 weeks. Both therapies significantly increased vaginal moisture, vaginal fluid volume, and vaginal elasticity.

Complementary Medicine

Acupuncture. A recent review indicated that approximately half of women experiencing menopause-associated symptoms use complementary and alternative medicine therapy instead of traditional therapies to manage their menopausal symptoms. One recent study reviewed the benefits of acupuncture on hot flashes.[60] The researchers reviewed 12 studies with 869 participants and found that acupuncture significantly reduced the frequency and severity of hot flashes on the Menopause-Specific Quality of Life questionnaire. So if you are aware of a good and qualified acupuncturist, it may be a treatment you want to consider.

Cognitive behavioral therapy (CBT). A number of complementary medicine approaches have been used to reduce the symptoms of menopause. These include acupuncture, yoga, tai chi, relaxation response, and others. All of them have provided some degree of success. At a plenary session of the North American Menopause Society annual meeting, all these approaches were compared, and all offered some benefit. However, the most consistently and best studied was a behavioral medicine approach that uses hypnotic relaxation therapy to reduce hot flashes; it is becoming popular and is considered as effective as other treatments for sleep problems and hot flashes.[61] The National Institutes of Health consensus and the American Academy of Sleep Medicine practice parameters recommend that cognitive behavioral therapy be considered standard treatment.

DR. GARY ELKINS is past president of the Society for Psychological Hypnosis. He is a professor in the department of psychology and neuroscience and also director of the Mind-Body Medicine Research Laboratory at Baylor University. Dr. Elkins is an accomplished scientist and author of *Relief from Hot Flashes: The Natural, Drug-Free Program to Reduce Hot Flashes, Improve Sleep, and Ease Stress.*

DR. MACHE SEIBEL: In your work, how big of a problem are hot flashes for menopausal women?

DR. GARY ELKINS: Most women will experience hot flashes at some time in their lives. Hot flashes are a particularly significant problem for women who have been diagnosed with breast cancer.

MS: All women are susceptible to hot flashes, but because women with breast cancer may get treatments that push them into menopause faster than going into menopause naturally, they suddenly have to deal with a life-threatening illness as well as hot flashes. And those are the very women who probably can't use estrogen.

GE: For women who slowly are going through menopause, the onset of hot flashes may be slower, but with medical or surgical treatments that rapidly reduce estrogen production, hot flashes can be sudden in onset and more severe.

MS: What is hypnotic relaxation therapy?

GE: Hypnotic relaxation refers to a state of consciousness involving a focus of attention, calm, and experiences that most people can relate to. For instance, when you go to a movie, you can suspend critical judgment during that time, and other things on your mind begin to fade into the background so you can remain absorbed in the movie experience. With hypnotic relaxation, a person learns how to enter into a deeply relaxed state, and then mental imagery is suggested for feeling cool or relaxed. The goal of *Relief from Hot Flashes* is to give women choices. One size does

(continued)

not fit all, especially when it comes to menopause treatments. Estrogen therapy is just one option. We discovered that women who used hypnotic relaxation therapy slept better and felt less stressful, and their overall quality of life and mood levels were higher. It is complementary to other medical treatments. In our most recent studies, we found that women on average reduced hot flashes by 80 percent! Some women had almost no hot flashes by the end of the program.

MS: That's a powerful tool. When women find life getting a bit out of control, for instance, they may be going through perimeno-pause, the window of up to 10 years before menopause and the year just beyond it, or they are struggling with sleep issues or stress because life can be pretty stressful independent of meno-pause, this method would be helpful. Can you explain how hyp-notic relaxation therapy works?

GE: The first step is to find a quiet place where you can sit with good support for your head, neck, and shoulders. Set aside 20 or 30 minutes of uninterrupted time. Some women practice first thing in the morning, while others prefer the end of the day before going to sleep. You will be entering a deeply relaxed state, so you want to be in a position where you can just let go, become limp and relaxed. I suggest sitting in a recliner, resting on a yoga mat, or lying on a bed with pillows. Close your eyes and begin to concentrate. Suggestions are given to imagine being in a favorite place, whether that's in the mountains or near the beach, just a place where you can imagine feeling very calmed. It can be a spe-cific place—a certain mountain vista or a specific cove on a beach—at a positive place or time in your memory.

Then you listen to audio recordings of the hypnotic relaxation sessions that are provided with the book. Each recording guides you mentally to a safe, pleasant place with images and recordings for coolness. Like walking down a path and feeling snow, or feeling a cool breeze off a lake that travels down the body. The more you practice, the more the audio recordings and techniques become familiar and natural. We've had some women who have gone through the program, relax so deeply, and feel so cool that they get goose bumps because they're so absorbed in the mental images.

MS: So 20 to 30 minutes every day for about 5 weeks and you'll be getting up to an 80 percent reduction in your hot flashes. Triggers for hot flashes include stress and sleep deprivation, and you're saying that most women who use hypnotic relaxation therapy will reduce their hot flashes and improve the quality of their lives.

GE: Yes, give it a chance. A mind-body therapy like this is something new, but as women become familiar with it, as they try it out, we found that most women love the benefits that occur within the first week or two.

Non-Estrogen Prescription Medications for Menopause

A few years ago no non-estrogen, approved prescription medications were available for the treatment of menopausal symptoms. There were only off-label uses of medications approved for other treatments. The observational uses of those medications let some drug developers do the necessary studies to gain approval for a new crop of menopausal treatments.

I mentioned Duavee earlier in this chapter. It is a new category of medication that combines an estrogen (Premarin) with an antiestrogen (bazedoxifene). Here are some of the other prescription non-estrogens that may be of help to you when estrogen isn't an option.

Antidepressants. In Chapter 6 we will discuss the impact of menopause on moodiness and menopause's association with depression. Depression affects at least one in four women aged 40 to 59. Moodiness and situational depression are so common in menopause that many women are prescribed antidepressants to help them through this transition. Once given antidepressants to deal with their emotions, many women observed and told their doctors that they had fewer hot flashes. That led to the off-label use of many selective serotonin reuptake inhibitors, or SSRIs, and testing of selective norepinephrine reuptake inhibitors (SNRIs) to see how effective they were for the treatment of hot flashes.

In June 2013, the FDA approved a low-dose version of the antidepressant paroxetine, known as Paxil, for women with moderate to severe hot flashes. The new medication is called Brisdelle, and it is the first nonhormonal treatment for hot flashes. The 7.5-milligram dosage is much less than the 30- to 40-milligram dose typically prescribed for the antidepressant Paxil, so it is not approved for treatment of depression. But for women with moderate to severe hot flashes who had seven or more daily, Brisdelle lowered the numbers by 57 to 59 percent. Though not as effective as estrogen, which will provide 65 to 80 percent reduction of hot flashes, Brisdelle is a real benefit to women who either can't or won't take HT. Some women taking this medication may have reported a reduction in sex drive, and it may increase risk of osteoporosis. Both of these should be discussed with your doctor.

The following antidepressant medications are still being used for symptoms of menopause, although they are not FDA approved for such purposes. If they work, they generally are effective within 2 to 4 weeks.

GENERIC NAME	BRAND NAME
escitalopram	Lexapro
fluoxetine	Prozac
paroxetine	Paxil
venlafaxine	Effexor

Ospemifene. Ospemifene is a class of medications called selective estrogen receptor modulators (SERMs) that is taken by mouth.[62] It is prescribed to women who have painful sex or drying and thinning of the vagina and vulva. (See page 154 for the discussion of atrophic vaginitis or vulvar atrophy, a genitourinary syndrome of menopause.) Ospemifene (Osphena) is available as 60-milligram tablets and can reduce painful intercourse, increase the pH of the vagina, increase the thickness of the vaginal walls, and improve vaginal moisture.

Some women who take this medication will have hot flashes, a vaginal discharge, and occasional muscle spasms. Osphena is not recommended for women who have a history of blood clots or stroke or a strong history of heart disease. If you are worried about taking estrogen or if you have an estrogen-sensitive cancer and treatment is causing vaginal dryness and painful sex, talk to your doctor about Osphena as an alternative treatment to estrogen. Visit EstrogenFixBook.com/resources to download a PDF summary sheet of non-estrogen prescription alternatives to keep as a reference.

Prasterone. On November 17, 2016, the FDA approved Intrarosa (prasterone), which contains the drug DHEA. This is a new intravaginal treatment for moderate to severe vaginal dryness and painful sex.[63] The once-daily intravaginal insert of a 6.5 mg suppository significantly improved painful sex, vaginal dryness, and thinning of the vaginal tissues. Although DHEA is included in some dietary supplements, none of those products have been tested for treating or preventing any disease.

The therapies for dealing with your symptoms may also fluctuate during this time. Perhaps taking evening primrose oil capsules was helpful until now, but your hot flashes are coming more frequently and with more intensity. If the time is right for you to start ET or EPT, then begin with the lowest dosage to see how you feel and react over the next 2 to 3 months. It's easiest to increase dosages until you reach the best dose for you. In most instances you'll reach an optimum dosage with just one increment. Many women experience large relief at the lowest dose. So why start at a higher dose? It's difficult, if not impossible, to know how much to reduce them.

Whether you choose ET, EPT, or an alternative therapy, keep in mind that the treatment of menopausal symptoms should start with making lifestyle changes. The four essential cornerstones of a healthy life before and after menopause are eating healthy whole foods, getting plenty of sleep at night, lowering your stress levels, and exercising regularly. In other words, to optimize menopause, you have to take care of the SUM of you, not just SOME of you. You'll find helpful information on making positive lifestyle changes throughout *The Estrogen Fix*. You can also find specific ways to turn these lifestyle cornerstones into midlife habits and create a menopause breakthrough. To see how your menopause symptoms compare to those of other women, visit www.MenopauseQuiz.com.

Chapter 4

The Estrogen Fix and Your Breasts

Even though heart disease is 10 times more likely than breast cancer to kill American women—heart disease kills one in every four females[1]—survey after survey and conversation after conversation with patients reveal that the majority of women believe they are more likely to die of breast cancer. Women view breast cancer as a double whammy—both life threatening and understandably life altering because of concern that the surgery and therapies to cure breast cancer could alter how they feel about themselves as women. There is no doubt that the fear of getting breast cancer from estrogen therapy is the main reason many women still look for an alternative to estrogen during menopause. But this is more than just fear; it has become a belief based on fear, and those types of beliefs are very difficult to change.

I get it. After the publication of the Women's Health Initiative study (WHI) in 2002 stated authoritatively that estrogen, and more specifically EPT, caused an increased risk of breast cancer, confusion and anxiety about safety caused use of both EPT and ET to plummet, not only in the United States[2] but also in Switzerland, Germany, Finland, and Australia.[3]

And more than a decade after the 2002 WHI study was reported and new understandings of the unfortunate errors in that seminal report have literally disproven and discredited some of the major findings of the original study, ET and EPT use in the United States remains low.

Why? Two words: breast cancer. According to two very senior research physicians in a July 2015 editorial in the journal *Menopause*, "Regarding risks associated with ET and EPT, breast cancer represents women's greatest concern." Worry about breast cancer is the major reason why women, and many of their doctors, are simply and emphatically saying NO to estrogen.[4, 5]

When the 2002 WHI study was discontinued, the participating women stopped taking EPT, but researchers continued to follow those women for an additional 12 years. During that time, most of EPT's benefits and risks reported in the 2002 WHI study faded. An exception was the risk of breast cancer. Following discontinuation of EPT, breast cancer risk did reduce each year, though a slight risk of breast cancer persisted.[6] How slight a risk? Less than one additional case of breast cancer diagnosed per 1,000 women who had formerly used EPT.

How significant is that? As mentioned in Chapter 3, it is approximately the same risk of getting breast cancer that comes from drinking one glass of wine daily and lower than the risk of drinking two glasses of wine daily. This outcome is very different from that of the women who took estrogen only (ET) and did not take a progestin with it. For them, the risk of breast cancer actually dropped significantly and was less than it was for the women taking a placebo.[7] In fact, in an article written in the *Journal of the National Cancer Institute*, Dr. Rowan Chlebowski, one of the main authors of the WHI reports and most vocal antiestrogen proponents, wrote that estrogen alone "statistically significantly decreased the risk of breast cancer."[8] He also said, "Currently, the different effects of estrogen plus progestin versus estrogen alone are not completely understood." Importantly, neither taking estrogen plus progestin nor taking estrogen alone increased the overall risk of dying according to this follow-up study.[9]

In a subsequent study that reanalyzed the original WHI data, those women who previously had taken HT before entering the WHI study and were then given EPT in the study had an increased risk of breast cancer. In contrast, EPT had no effect on those women who had never taken HT prior to receiving EPT in the WHI.[10] This is an important nuance because most women who start EPT have not taken HT in the past.

More recently, a study of 489,105 women evaluated the risk of breast cancer death among women who had taken HT.[11] In general, breast cancer is fatal in 1 in 10 women. But women who used HT for any length of time before developing breast cancer had a 1 in 20 risk of dying or half as much. This is very important information for women considering HT.

The real shame is that many women and many doctors still do not realize that the risks of taking estrogen are so much less than originally thought and the benefits are so much greater. ET lowers the risk of breast cancer and EPT does not increase the risk of dying from breast cancer. Knowing this, plus understanding your estrogen window, is a game changer for deciding whether or not to take estrogen. It's also important to realize that low-dose vaginal estrogens were not studied in the WHI reports, nor were there any breast cancer or other serious risks associated with taking them. In fact, in Finland, vaginal estrogen is available in drug stores without prescription. Yet after the initial findings of the 2002 WHI report were made public, a black-box warning was required to be placed on the package inserts of all estrogens—including vaginal estrogens—that included all the safety concerns of the 2002 study, which adds to women's concerns and anxiety.[12] All this flies in the face of the fact that right up to the publication of the 2002 WHI study, which created the belief that estrogen was a cause of breast cancer, a number of publications reported that high doses of estrogen are actually effective *treatment* for advanced metastatic breast cancer.[13]

Many menopause experts, like myself, and clinical researchers like Dr. Richard Santen at the University of Virginia, don't believe that estrogen was the cause of breast cancers in most of the women who participated in the WHI studies.[14] The fact is that if estrogen did cause cancer, it would take approximately 10 years for a clinically detectable tumor to appear. Remember that the WHI study was halted just after 5 years. The likelihood is that if estrogen did play a role, it would be to unmask an existing breast cancer rather than cause it.

How the Body's Estrogen Affects the Breasts at Different Ages

Throughout a woman's life, the estrogen produced naturally by her body has an effect on her breasts, causing them to change throughout much of her life span. By this I mean that the cells of breast tissue continue to mature from before puberty until well into adulthood. To

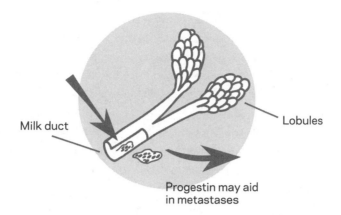

Milk duct

Lobules

Progestin may aid
in metastases

explain this better, we need to take a closer look at the anatomy of a breast. Each breast contains 15 to 20 lobes that are comprised of groups of lobules that are the milk-producing glands. These lobules are connected together by breast tissue, blood vessels, and ducts.

If we take an even closer look at each of the lobules, we will find 10 to 100 rounded alveoli that open into the smallest branches of the milk ducts. These small branches join together to form larger ducts that end in the terminal, or lactiferous, ducts. Early in puberty, when estrogen is just starting to be produced but before ovulation and progesterone production begins, the ducts of the breasts begin to increase and branch. Later in puberty ovulation begins, and with it, the production of progesterone, which stimulates the alveolar cells to start developing. Without progesterone, these changes do not occur.

When a young woman enters her reproductive years, she develops regular menstrual cycles, causing the tips (called the terminal end buds) of the ducts, but not the bases, to divide more rapidly. Because the terminal end buds are the least mature terminal ductal structures, they are the ones most susceptible to carcinogens.[15] These terminal end buds are the growing fringes of the mammary gland, and they are undifferentiated. With each menstrual cycle, some of the terminal end buds mature (differentiate), as do the lobules. Know that the more mature or differentiated a cell is, the more resistant it is to developing cancer.

From this time forward until menopause, the breasts are in a constant state of change with each menstrual cycle. Over time, the terminal end buds and lobules (which early in puberty, before the first menstrual cycle, are called type I lobules) become increasingly differentiated. They progress to type II lobules. When women receive hormonal stimulation or become pregnant, they differentiate further to type III lobules. The most differentiated lobules, type IV, are only found in women who have been pregnant. This is why women who have had a full-term pregnancy early in life are four times *less* likely to develop breast cancer than women who do not get pregnant.[16]

All these changes in the breasts explain why mammograms are not always 100 percent accurate. Mammograms sometimes suggest a cancer when there isn't one (false-positive result) and fail to see one when a cancer actually is there (false-negative result).[17] According to the *Journal of the National Cancer Institute,* "almost a quarter of all women who regularly underwent screening mammograms over a 10-year period received a false-positive result from at least one of their exams."[18] Women who take EPT are at more risk of a false-positive exam. Adding ultrasound of the breasts to the mammograms seems to be effective for distinguishing between cancerous and noncancerous cysts because it can detect the greater bloodflow associated with cancer. Ultrasound alone isn't very effective because it can't detect the calcium deposits that are one of the earliest signs of breast cancer.[19]

Women's breasts are denser when they are younger and more hormones are naturally present. About 75 percent of premenopausal women have dense breasts.[20] After menopause, estrogen and progesterone levels are lower and there is less cell division in the breasts. Both the ducts and the alveolar tissue become less active and the breasts become smaller as the tips of the ducts, not the bases, shrink in size. Only about 25 percent of women in menopause have dense breasts. The cells of the breast, however, "remember" estrogen and progesterone, and if they are exposed to these hormones later in life, they respond quickly and enlarge again. This does not mean that these changes are equivalent to causing cancer; it does mean that EPT will cause the changes that occurred naturally between puberty and menopause to resume, which makes the breasts denser.

After menopause, if EPT is not taken, the breasts change as fat replaces the denser tissue. These changes allow mammograms to see into the breasts of postmenopausal women not on EPT more easily than into the breasts of premenopausal women.[21] As you have probably already guessed, EPT stimulates the already-sensitized breast tissue to become denser, fuller, and larger.[22] From a practical point of view, about

40 percent of women who take EPT will have denser breasts while taking the combined estrogen/progestogen regimen compared with only 2 percent of women taking estrogen only either orally or transdermally.[23] This increased density may include the entire breast, several small areas, or one specific area.

The question is, does taking EPT increase your risk of undetected breast cancer because the radiologist can't see the cancer? In a study of nearly 330,000 women between the ages of 40 and 89, mammograms remained accurate in detecting breast cancer.[24] In general, the study found, the accuracy of mammograms increases as women's breasts become fattier and less dense with age. This means that mammograms are more accurate beyond menopause, whether or not the women are using hormone therapy. The difference was that women using HT who had denser breasts sometimes needed additional studies like another mammogram or ultrasound to confirm whether or not cancer was present. So EPT doesn't increase your risk of breast cancer because of a radiologist error, but you may require additional testing.

Benign breast masses, including fibroadenomas and cysts (so-called fibrocystic disease or lumpy breasts) also become more common[25] in menopausal women. All these changes make mammograms more difficult for the radiologist to read, and as mentioned above, additional mammograms, ultrasounds, and even biopsies may be called for. Once the EPT is discontinued, the radiologists' ability to read a mammogram is the same as for women who have never been on EPT.[26] Selective estrogen receptor modulators, or SERMs, are estrogen-like hormones that have been modified to act like estrogen on the bones and like an anti-estrogen on the breasts. Two examples are raloxifene (a common drug for osteoporosis) and tamoxifen (a common drug to treat breast cancer). Once we realize that estrogen and progestogen have an effect on breast tissue and that the specific effects change at different points of the life cycle, it is easy to understand how scientific studies on the effect of EPT on the breasts can quickly become confusing.

Estrogen and the BRCA Gene Mutation

You have likely heard about the BRCA or BReast CAncer gene.[27] There are two varieties: BRCA1 and BRCA2. A mutation, which is an abnormal change, in this gene significantly increases a woman's lifetime risk of developing breast or ovarian cancer. When I first found out about this gene, my wife, Sharon, got tested immediately because she has lost so many of the women in her family to ovarian cancer. Sharon was positive for the BRCA2 gene mutation.

The BRCA gene isn't the main cause of breast cancer. Only about 5 to 10 percent of breast cancers are due to known genetic mutations.[28] But having this mutation can have a major impact on the person with the mutation and her family (men can also have the BRCA gene mutation). Compared with the normal risk of breast cancer, which is 12 percent over the lifetime, a woman with BRCA1 mutations has about a 55 to 65 percent risk of developing breast cancer, and women who inherit the BRCA2 mutation have about a 45 percent chance of developing breast cancer by age 70.[29]

While about 1.3 percent of women in general will develop ovarian cancer in their lifetime, a little fewer than 15 percent of ovarian cancers are linked to mutated genes. Women with BRCA1 mutations have a 39 percent risk and women with BRCA2 have an 11 to 17 percent risk of developing ovarian cancer by age 70. This is a huge increase in risk of cancer for these women—one that carries a 50 percent risk that their children, both male and female, will inherit the gene from them and also be at risk of these increases in cancer (men have increased risk of prostate cancer). Note that having the BRCA gene mutation is only an increase in the *chance* of getting cancer; it does not mean that a woman with that gene will absolutely develop cancer.

One of the most famous people with a BRCA gene mutation is actress and humanitarian Angelina Jolie, who very bravely and publicly wrote about and discussed having the BRCA1 gene mutation and a strong family history of cancer. She had both of her breasts removed prophetically in 2013 to lower her risk of breast cancer. Given her young age of 37, this had to be a huge and difficult decision. Ms. Jolie then underwent additional surgery[30] to remove her fallopian tubes and ovaries (her uterus was not removed) to lower her risk of ovarian cancer because her mother died from that disease at age 56. I know firsthand from my wife Sharon's experience that this must have been a challenging, well-thought-out decision, because surgically removing both ovaries put Ms. Jolie into what is medically called "surgical menopause."

I applaud Angelina Jolie for her courageous and open discussion of her BRCA1 gene screening and the actions she took to lower her risk of breast and ovarian cancers. She has raised the issue of heredity and cancer awareness for millions of women and given them the courage to discuss openly the benefits of genetic testing. I also applaud her for how well she worked together with her doctors to figure out how to work through her complex and challenging situation and create a collaborative treatment plan. She figured out how to remove the tissue in danger of developing cancer and how to immediately put into place an estrogen plan as she entered her estrogen window to help retain her libido and lower her risk of hip fracture, heart disease, and dementia.[31] I want to expand upon a few additional points that could make Ms. Jolie's brave public disclosure even more impactful.

The first is that BRCA, particularly the BRCA2 gene mutation, is associated with an up to 5 times greater likelihood of developing pancreatic cancer. Pancreatic cancer is on the rise and likely to overtake breast cancer and replace colon cancer as the number-two cause of death due to cancer by 2020.[32] People with BRCA, and in particular BRCA2, should have this discussion with their doctors. Again, I learned this firsthand. Sharon dodged the breast and ovarian cancer bullets but developed pancreatic cancer. Now 5 years out she is thankfully disease-free. Being screened for pancreatic cancer is not theoretical.

The second point is that Ms. Jolie stated that she took transdermal estrogen. Because her ovaries were surgically removed, she was in early menopause. That she took estrogen is an important point to underscore, because going into menopause before age 46 and *not* taking estrogen in early or premature menopause is associated with up to a 70 percent increase risk of Alzheimer's disease, a 23 percent increased risk of heart disease, a 28 percent increased risk of premature death, an 80 percent increased risk of Parkinson's disease, and potentially an increased risk of breast cancer that is prevented if estrogen is taken at the time of surgical menopause and at least through the age of natural menopause.[33, 34, 35, 36] Note that women with BRCA who choose to take estrogen do not appear to be at any increased risk of breast cancer compared to women with BRCA not taking estrogen.[37] Taking estrogen will also help Ms. Jolie maintain her youthful looks.

The third point is that Ms. Jolie was prescribed a progesterone-secreting IUD. I talked about this in Chapter 3 as a way to minimize the risk of taking progestogen if you have your uterus. As a result, she can take estrogen without having to take oral progestogen, which is otherwise required to protect her uterine lining from cancer. The take-home message: Women who are on estrogen and who still have their uterus can talk with their doctors about the option of using a progesterone-secreting IUD off-label as a possible alternative to oral progesterone.[38]

The BRCA gene test is a blood or saliva test offered only to women who are likely to have an inherited mutation, based on personal or family history, or who have specific types of breast cancer.

Lifestyle Tips for Breast Health

- Maintain a healthy weight and lifestyle. The greater your weight, the greater your risk of breast cancer.

- Limit alcohol. Drink alcohol in moderation—no more than one 4-ounce glass several times a week.

- Quit smoking. It can't be said enough times. Cigarette smoking affects every aspect of your health and wellness. That includes an increased risk of breast cancer among smokers. The rate of new cases was 24 percent higher in smokers than in nonsmokers and 13 percent higher in former smokers than in nonsmokers.[39] According to the American Cancer Society, the earlier you begin smoking, the higher your risk of invasive breast cancer. Women who began smoking before their first menstrual period had a 61 percent higher risk than women who never smoked; those who started smoking after their first cycle, but 11 or more years before having a child, had a 45 percent higher risk.

- Move your body. Whether it's walking, swimming, Zumba, cycling, or any other aerobic exercise, the more you move, the better. A study of previously inactive postmenopausal women had two groups of women do moderate to vigorous exercise for 1 year.[40] The scores—weight loss, fitness, and all-over health—were higher for the women who exercised 300 minutes per week than for those who exercised just 150 minutes

The BRCA gene test currently is not routinely performed on women at average risk of breast and ovarian cancers; however, in an interview I had with Susan M. Domchek, MD, who is the executive director of the Basser Center for BRCA at the University of Pennsylvania, the discussion has begun on whether or not we should be testing all women of Jewish descent.

per week, especially for obese women. "These results suggest additional benefit of higher-volume aerobic exercise for adiposity outcomes and possibly a lower risk of postmenopausal breast cancer." And for women who do develop breast cancer, exercising for at least 30 minutes daily has been shown to lower the risk of recurrence.[41]

• Know your family history. If any women—or men, for that matter—have had breast cancer, let your health-care provider know. That includes your mother, sisters, aunts, grandmothers, and first cousins. Because ovarian cancer and colon cancer are also linked to breast cancer through some genetic deletions such as BRCA, a history of those cancers or even pancreatic cancer may suggest a need for genetic screening; again, tell your family cancer history to your health-care provider.

• Perform a breast self-exam. Every woman should do a visual and manual breast self-examination monthly.[42] If you notice a lump, flattening, or indentation in the breast or armpit, pain or tenderness, or discharge from or change in the nipples, make an appointment to see your doctor immediately. At your annual physical examination, your health-care provider will perform a thorough breast examination as well. Every woman should have an annual mammogram after the age of 40. If you have a family history of breast cancer, then mammograms are recommended at an earlier age.

Talking to My Patients about Estrogen and Breast Cancer

When my patients and I talk about estrogen therapy, they ask many questions, including "If I take estrogen, will it increase my chances of getting breast cancer? Is it right for me? Can I take it? For how long? What kind of estrogen is best for me?" Given that most women who avoid EPT do so because of fears related to breast cancer, this line of questioning isn't surprising. Imagine the relief they feel once they know they don't have to choose between estrogen and breast cancer.

Every person is different, not only medically but also emotionally. No one approach or therapy applies to everyone in the same ways, and I share some basic guidelines with my patients who are dealing with the symptoms of menopause and individualize beyond that. Because your situation is unique, it's best that you talk with your health-care provider about an individual approach for you. What you choose to do may vary depending on your genetic, family, and recent medical histories. My hope is that with the information you've gained in *The Estrogen Fix*, your decision will be based on accurate facts and not myth-information. I'll share more with you about taking estrogen in Chapter 10.

Chapter 5

The Estrogen Fix and Your Heart

If you are like many of my patients, you worry more about developing breast cancer than heart disease. You're trying to figure out how to deal with hot flashes, lower libido, pants that are too tight, or getting a good night's sleep. Whether estrogen is good or bad for your heart may not be at the top of your thoughts. If you do think about heart disease, it's probably in relation to your mother or other older family members.

But as I mentioned in Chapter 4, as a woman, you are 10 times more likely to die of heart disease than of breast cancer. Understanding your estrogen window and the differences between ET and EPT can add years to your life and impact the quality of it.

The message about estrogen's role in heart disease has been confusing, to say the least. During my career in medicine, I've watched the pendulum swing back and forth and back again from estrogen considered effective in preventing heart disease to estrogen thought to increase the risk of heart disease to estrogen once again beneficial against heart disease. This chapter explains that if you want to protect your heart from disease, you must know about your estrogen window.

It's hard to imagine it, but for more than a century, heart disease was thought to happen only to men. Doctors actually believed that women didn't suffer from heart disease and almost never had heart attacks. It's another example of poorly designed studies impacting public and medical perceptions about women's health. The initial studies were done well more than 100 years ago, when the average age of death for women was before the age of menopause. The autopsy studies done to find heart disease in women didn't find any because the women autopsied died before the age of menopause, which is when most women begin to develop heart disease.

Fast-forward 150 years and heart disease—not breast or any other cancer—is the number-one killer of women over age 65 and the second leading cause of death among women aged 45 to 64. Women account for 52 percent of the 80 million Americans who have heart disease and *who die from heart disease and heart attacks*. More women die from cardiovascular disease than from all other causes of death such as lung cancer, breast cancer, stroke, and COPD (chronic obstructive pulmonary disease) combined.[1] It's really important to discover what you can do to protect your heart and not allow misinformation to cloud your beliefs, because more women than men have died of heart disease since the mid-1980s.

That's why the information in this chapter is so important. Beliefs are often hard to change both for women and for the doctors who treat them. Despite the statistics, it is still difficult for many women with cardiac disease to receive proper diagnosis and treatment. Women, and even some doctors, need to be informed about the possible benefits of taking ET during their estrogen window, if not just for its long-lasting cardioprotective effects. EPT offers significant relief of menopausal symptoms, and it does so without increasing cardiac risk if taken in the estrogen window.

I recognize that even with the current thinking, some doctors don't feel estrogen is beneficial in preventing heart disease. That's not surprising. Information on the risks and benefits of ET and EPT has been confusing and contradictory through the years. In the 1990s, recommending that women take estrogen was standard, and 90 percent of premenopausal women who had had a hysterectomy were prescribed ET because the observational data suggested that it protected them from heart disease.[2] In fact, the benefits of estrogen on the female heart are believed to be why atherosclerosis and heart disease appears to lag 10 years or more in premenopausal women than age-matched men.[3]

During the 1990s, hysterectomies were performed on nearly 600,000 women in the United States each year; that's 12 every 10 minutes.[4, 5] Fifty-two percent of all hysterectomies were performed on women aged 44 years or younger. Unless those women take estrogen, they are at significantly increased risk of heart disease.[6] Ninety percent of the women who were in their fifties or younger and who had hysterectomies in the 1990s were prescribed estrogen for 4 to 5 years. There was even a period of time when estrogen was considered so good at protecting against heart disease that it was given to men, including those who had suffered heart attacks. But as you might expect, the men with a history of heart attack didn't do well on estrogen. In fact, many died after taking it for a while.

To prove whether or not estrogen prevented heart disease, there were two Women's Health Initiative (WHI) studies. In one, women who had their uterus were given either a placebo or Prempro, a pill that combined the conjugated estrogen Premarin plus a progestin. Progestin is a synthetic chemical that sometimes acts like progesterone, but it has a slightly different chemical structure. The progestin was necessary for women who still had their uterus because they were at high risk of developing uterine cancer if taking estrogen only for a prolonged number of years. When women who have their uterus take estrogen plus progestogen (EPT) for at least 10 days of each month, uterine cancer virtually never occurs.

The second WHI study was simultaneously conducted for women who had their uterus removed by hysterectomy. Since their uterus had been removed, these women didn't need to take progestin, so they were given either estrogen only (ET) in the form of Premarin or a placebo. The age range of the women in both groups was 50 to 79 with most of the treated women being aged 60 to 79 and the placebo group mostly aged 50 to 59.

The first WHI study results on EPT were published in July 2002[7] and included findings about prescribing women a placebo or Premarin plus Provera (Prempro). The study found that women who took the combination of estrogen plus a progestin had a higher risk of heart disease, breast cancer, blood clots, and strokes than women who took a placebo. That same group of women who took Prempro was also found to have a *lower* risk both of breaking hips and of colon cancer, findings that were almost never discussed.

When these negative findings were released, the study was immediately canceled ahead of schedule because the findings sounded so terrible and dangerous. Taking estrogen plus progestin was viewed as toxic, and the media went wild. Each day a new headline regaled the dangers of "estrogen." Women felt betrayed by the medical establishment for giving them a harmful medicine, and they immediately wanted to stop taking any estrogen-containing medication, a belief that persists today. Prescriptions for Premarin and Prempro, which contain the two female hormones, dropped 73 percent from 67.2 million in 2000 to 18.5 million in 2006, according to a press release. More than 5,000 lawsuits have been filed against Wyeth, the company that manufactured the pills, alleging its hormones caused cancer.[8]

It's understandable. Imagine a prevention study on a medicine that was supposed to protect your heart gets prematurely halted because that very medicine turned out to increase risk of breast cancer, heart attack, stroke, and other undesirable outcomes. That was the takeaway. There was palpable tension, confusion, and fear.

I vividly remember my office phone ringing off the hook with literally hundreds of women worried that they too would develop those diseases or complications. The situation wasn't helped by the fact that the media often referred to Prempro as hormone therapy or HT and sometimes just as estrogen. As a result, women and their doctors generalized the study's EPT findings to ET and every other medication containing estrogen.

Within 18 months, half the women in the United States who were using estrogen stopped taking it,[9] including almost two million women who had no uterus and were using only estrogen (ET) and not using the Prempro (EPT) study drug that also contained a progestin.

Later the WHI looked at the effects of taking just estrogen on women who had no uterus. In that study the researchers found that women aged 50 to 59 years taking ET did not have an increased risk of heart disease; they had a *reduced* risk of heart disease.[10] A later follow-up analysis of the estrogen-alone study published in 2011[11] found that the total risk of death was reduced by 13 per 10,000 women per year, mostly because of decreased heart disease, although there was also a lower risk of cancer and other causes of death. More recently, a paper I mentioned in Chapter 4 that studied 489,105 women who were given estrogen or estrogen plus a progestogen found that the risk of dying from coronary heart disease was reduced by 19 fewer women per 1,000 women and the risk of dying from stroke was reduced by 7 per 1,000 women[12] if they started taking it during their estrogen window. The estrogen used in that study was almost entirely estradiol in dosages of 1 to 2 milligrams daily. The same researchers in another study also found that women under the age of 60 who discontinue their postmenopausal HT have an increased risk of death from heart attack and stroke within the first year of stopping compared to women who continued HT treatment.[13] This was not the case for women who discontinued HT after age 60.

The distressing thing was that despite the later positive findings, the impact of the initial 2002 study continued to have a negative effect, and the number of estrogen prescriptions continued to decline[14] for all types of medications that contained estrogen. You know how hard it is to fix a damaged reputation. So it was for estrogen; it was difficult, if not impossible, to remove a fear that had bored its way into the subconscious of a society.

Lipid and Cholesterol Levels in Women

Lipids are fat-like substances in the blood and body tissues. Cholesterol is the main lipid, and it's made up of different parts, such as HDL, LDL, and triglycerides, that I'll talk about more shortly. Most people worry about their cholesterol levels. Nearly 100 million people take a cholesterol-lowering drug,[15] and since the criteria for taking them were changed in November 2013,[16] that number rapidly increasing. Suffice it to say, with so many people taking these medications, you probably know that controlling cholesterol levels is important and that an increase of cholesterol is associated with heart disease. You might think that in general, cholesterol is bad.

Cholesterol, like most things, is not inherently entirely good or bad. Our bodies need cholesterol to insulate nerve cells in the brain and to create structure for the walls of cells. Cholesterol is also a basic molecule in the production of many of the body's hormones. Seventy-five percent of cholesterol is made either by the liver or cells elsewhere in the body. The other 25 percent comes from food.

Like butter or vegetable shortening, cholesterol is a fat, and it doesn't dissolve in the blood. To be transported throughout the body—fat and water don't mix, and your body is mostly water—cholesterol attaches to proteins, and it's the proteins that circulate in the blood vessels. Since this molecule is a combination of a protein and fat or lipid, it is called a lipoprotein. One type is HDL, or high-density lipoprotein. HDL is sometimes called good cholesterol because it is believed to mop up LDL from the blood vessel walls and remove it from the body. LDL, or low-density lipoprotein, is called lousy or bad cholesterol because it can build up in the walls of arteries and cause plaque that can narrow blood vessels and reduce bloodflow.

The plaque forms because LDL at higher levels can be absorbed into the artery walls and attract white blood cells (WBCs). The WBCs act like Pac-Men and eat the fatty particles to try and heal the blood vessel, but it doesn't work well. Instead, inflammation and fatty deposits called plaque form and cause the blood vessels to stiffen and narrow. That, in turn, reduces bloodflow, increases blood pressure, and causes the heart to pump harder to push blood through the narrower, harder arteries. Eventually that can lead to chest pain, stroke, heart attack, and many other symptoms, depending on where the plaque forms. If you add extra body weight to lots of plaque, the pump you call your heart then has to pump blood through a narrower set of pipes to more pounds. That's a lot of extra work for your pump.

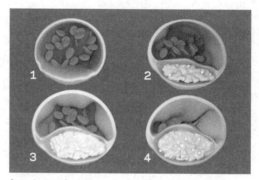

Arteries, with progressively increasing amounts of plaque.

It's also important to point out that different forms of LDL and HDL differ in how harmful or how protective they are.[17] According to Dr. Steven Masley in his book *The 30-Day Heart Tune-Up*, LDL cholesterol can be small and dense or big and fluffy. The fluffy variety is packed with nutrients and carries fat-soluble vitamins and antioxidants to your cells. It's the smaller LDL particles that are the problem; they cause plaque to grow, and that is believed to be because of their smaller size, which makes it easier for them to penetrate the lining cells of arteries.

LDL can be influenced by behavior. The more you stay physically active; eat fruits, vegetables, and healthy fats like unsaturated fats and omega-3s; and avoid refined carbohydrates and saturated and trans fats, the less small LDL you'll have. Although oral estrogen is consistently found to lower the total levels of cholesterol and total LDL levels, only some studies suggest estrogen also helps to lower small LDL particles, while others suggest that oral estrogen increases small LDL particles.[18, 19]

In contrast, transdermal estrogen has little effect on either total LDL or HDL levels but does slightly decrease total plasma triglyceride levels and produce larger LDL particles that are resistant to oxidation, which is a good thing.[20]

HDL also comes in two sizes: HDL2, which is big and able to remove LDL and other negatives from the arteries, and HDL3, which is smaller and not very effective at removing the bad stuff from your arteries. So size does matter. Estrogen may play a role in increasing the HDL2 subfractions.[21]

While the typical blood tests for HDL and LDL are accurate 80 percent of the time, according to Dr. Masley, that means they aren't precise at predicting heart disease 20 percent of the time. If you are at high risk of heart disease, ask your doctor to check an advanced lipid profile.

So what role does estrogen play in heart disease in addition to influencing cholesterol levels? The walls of blood vessels have estrogen receptors where estrogen can have a direct impact. A particularly large number of estrogen receptors are in the blood vessels of the heart, the aorta, and the saphenous vein, which is a large vein in the legs. When estrogen attaches to these receptors, it activates certain genetic activity that helps these blood vessels dilate and improves the flow of calcium ions, which enhances bloodflow and has other beneficial actions.[22, 23] In laboratory studies done with arteries taken from menopausal women not taking estrogen, the arteries were found to function poorly. When estrogen was added to the culture dishes, the function of the arteries improved.[24] In a study involving estrogen given to women after menopause, the women's blood vessels responded to estradiol with the most dilation and improved bloodflow if the women were within 5 years of menopause.[25] All this information points to the role that estrogen has on bloodflow in women and highlights the importance of taking advantage of your estrogen window for overall optimum health benefits. The closer to the beginning of menopause you start taking estrogen, the greater estrogen's potential benefit to your heart.

The Estrogen Fix and Your Coronary Arteries

In Chapter 6 you will read about estrogen's positive effect on the inner walls of blood vessels, increasing nitric oxide levels, which opens blood vessels, lowering cytokines and other inflammatory substances, and keeping the blood vessels in your brain more flexible. The same is true in the blood vessels of your heart.

Before menopause, women have lower LDL cholesterol levels and higher HDL cholesterol levels than men of the same age.[26] Things change after menopause when estrogen levels are lower; LDL cholesterol levels rise and often are greater than the levels of age-matched men. In addition, the LDL particles shift to smaller, denser sizes, which are more likely to cause atherosclerosis. Estrogen, particularly estrogen taken by mouth, also has a major impact on cholesterol levels in women. It reduces LDL cholesterol levels and increases HDL cholesterol levels in postmenopausal women with normal or increased baseline values.[27] This is due to the "first-pass effect" of the liver.

Here's how the first-pass effect works and why it matters here. Estrogen taken orally is absorbed from the gut and enters the blood circulation after first passing through the liver, which in many ways acts as a processing center for what comes through your mouth. This first-pass effect is responsible for many of the good and the bad effects of estrogen. If you tap a liver vein after swallowing an oral dose of estrogen, the concentration of estrogen in the liver will be 12 times higher than blood levels after the estrogen gets metabolized, so the cells of the liver are exposed to 12 times more estrogen than other cells of the body are.

The liver has many responsibilities, and among them are involvement in how the body metabolizes sugars and fats and how it synthesizes blood-clotting factors. So taking estrogen orally will increase HDL cholesterol and lower LDL cholesterol, which are both positive things in terms of preventing heart disease. Oral estrogen will also have beneficial effects on blood glucose levels. Unfortunately, the first-pass effect of oral estrogen can increase the concentration of blood-clotting factors that are made in the liver. That is why oral estrogen can increase the risk of blood clots and stroke.

Because estrogen taken through the skin (transdermally) or vagina is absorbed directly into the bloodstream and skips the first pass through the liver, any non-oral route of taking estrogen avoids the first-pass effect, so it has no effect on LDL and HDL levels and it doesn't increase the risk of blood clots.[28] This means that if you have a history of liver disease you should avoid oral estrogen, and if you are worried about the risk of blood clots, non-oral routes will be less prone to cause that problem.

In one study where estrogen was infused into the left coronary arteries of the hearts of 20 postmenopausal women, the investigators felt that most of the benefits of estrogen on the heart were on the microcirculation.[29] As explained elsewhere in this chapter, women who have heart attacks typically have disease of the small microvessels of the heart rather than the large coronary arteries. Women also have 10 times more estrogen receptors than men, which allows estrogen to dilate their arteries more than can occur in men. Men, on the other hand, tend to have blockage in their large coronary arteries. That is a major reason why women's symptoms of heart attack often differ from men's and why the typical tests used to diagnose heart disease in men often aren't helpful to diagnose heart disease in women.[30] It's also why not taking estrogen during the estrogen window deprives women of the dilating effects of estrogen on their heart's microcirculation.

Dr. Phil Sarrel of Yale shared a story with me of a patient who illustrates estrogen's ability to dilate the arteries of the heart.

Kirstin was 46 when her uterus was removed because of uterine fibroids. The doctor also removed her fallopian tubes and ovaries at the same time. She began having severe hot flashes and chest pain almost immediately. Worried about her heart, she went to see a cardiologist who took her history, did some evaluations, and determined that she did not have heart disease; because the hot flashes happened at the same time as the chest pain, he felt the chest pain was due to the sudden drop of estrogen caused by removal of her ovaries.

Kirstin was very early in her estrogen window and was prescribed a transdermal estradiol patch. Both her hot flashes and her chest pain stopped within 1 week. The estrogen prevented her coronary arteries from narrowing, and that stopped her chest pain.

Why Is It So Difficult to Diagnose Heart Disease in Women?

Women and many doctors aren't fully aware of how many women have undetected heart disease. They should be. According to the American Heart Association, 35,000 American women under 50 years of age have heart attacks each year, and an overall increase of heart attacks among women is seen about 10 years after menopause.[31]

Among the many differences between men and women is how they experience heart disease or heart attack symptoms. For instance, if I asked you what the symptoms of a heart attack are, which is when the bloodflow that brings oxygen to the heart is severely reduced or stopped, you'd probably answer "crushing chest pain or radiating pain down the left, sometimes the right, arm, and cold sweats." While those symptoms are common in men and may occur in women, women are

WHEN 49-year-old Martha was referred to me as a new patient, she told me she had had a heart attack during the previous year. She was at home, racing around to get her kids off to school and getting dinner ready for that evening before she left for work. Suddenly she began to sweat and felt so uncharacteristically tired and light-headed that she had to lie down on the floor to gather herself. She felt nauseated and had an upset stomach.

When her friend Sue luckily happened to stop by, she took one look at Martha and said, "Why don't you call an ambulance?" Martha responded that she had planned to do that as soon as she finished cleaning up the kitchen; she didn't want the EMTs to come in and see her house looking like a mess. Really.

I have heard similar stories a number of times and wrote about it in my book *Save Your Life: What to Do in a Medical Emergency*. If you ever start to feel like you're not yourself and experience any of the symptoms mentioned above, call 911 immediately, unlock the front door, and sit or lie down until the EMTs arrive.

First, if you do have persistent symptoms like chest pain, shortness of breath, extreme fatigue, back or jaw pain, or any of the others described above, tell your health-care provider as soon as possible. For women, the best way to detect heart disease is to have an exercise stress test and a stress echocardiogram. These tests involve walking on a treadmill or pedaling a stationary bike for 5 to 10 minutes at increasing levels of difficulty while your blood pressure and heart rate are monitored. Your doctor can then determine how your heart specifically responds to exertion to see if there is adequate bloodflow to it. If your physician detects any problems, then an angiogram may be the next step, but the best test for diagnosing microvascular heart disease is still being figured out.

more likely to feel profound fatigue, lightheadedness, dizziness, nausea, and vomiting. They may also notice neck, jaw, back, or upper abdominal pain. They may complain of an upset stomach. When women do experience heart attack–related chest pain, it often lasts more than 10 minutes and sometimes longer than 30 minutes. This is called microvascular angina.

Female heart attack patients frequently describe their symptoms as flu-like. Some also complain of sleep problems, fatigue, and lack of energy, which can be confusing because they are also symptoms of menopause. Fewer than half of the women who have heart attacks will have the classic crushing chest pain, which is one of the main reasons many women don't realize they are having a heart attack. Even when women go to the emergency room, the diagnosis often goes undetected.

Sometimes the standard tests for heart disease aren't helpful either. For example, heart disease is often diagnosed through an angiogram, in which a small catheter is placed through an artery and threaded into the larger heart arteries. A small amount of a dye is injected to see if the arteries are blocked. If there is a blockage, a stent, or a tube, is placed in the blocked artery passage to open the blockage. More than 50 percent of women who get a catheterization will have no blockage found, but they still have persistent chest pain and tenacious symptoms. Many are then falsely reassured that they don't have heart disease, when in fact they do. It's easy to imagine that if you go to the hospital thinking you're having a heart attack and are then told your heart is fine, you'll be much less likely to go back to the emergency room should the same symptoms reoccur.

Why does this happen? Because in women the disease is often in the small arteries of the heart instead of the larger ones, where it tends to occur in men. This is the microvascular disease or microvascular dysfunction mentioned previously; the larger arteries are fine, but all the smaller blood vessels are affected. And that causes the different symptoms in women.

Microvascular disease occurs because women are generally smaller in height and weight than men. As a result, women's arteries are also smaller than those of men, and the fat builds up differently in their blood vessels. According to the American Heart Association, women who have lower than normal estrogen levels at any point in their lives are at risk of microvascular heart disease. Low estrogen levels before menopause put women at higher risk of microvascular disease. Remember, once women stop making estrogen, they are no longer stimulating the estrogen receptors in the arteries of their heart to dilate and bring extra bloodflow to their hearts. That lower bloodflow increases their risk of heart disease.

Microvascular disease can't be treated with angioplasty or other types of surgery. Treatment is all about making lifestyle changes—diet to reduce cholesterol, exercise, stress reduction, getting enough sleep, not smoking—to reduce the underlying issues that contribute to microvascular disease.

Menopause and Heart Disease

Menopause does not cause heart disease per se. A decline in the amount of estrogen menopausal women produce may be one factor for heart disease and may contribute to microvascular heart disease, but diet, level of fitness, weight, smoking, and other lifestyle issues play equally important roles. Estrogen is believed to play a role in keeping calcium deposits from building up in arteries, which may explain why the rate of heart attacks increases in women 10 years after menopause. Along these lines, if you look over the results of the famous Framingham Heart Study, you'll see there were no heart disease deaths in premenopausal women in the entire study. Within 10 years after menopause, however, the numbers of deaths from heart disease in women were the same as they were in men. Once again this shows the impact of menopause on heart disease.

Women who go through menopause before age 46 have twice the likelihood of having coronary heart disease and stroke as women who go into menopause at a later age, and this risk is independent of a woman's ethnic background or other traditional cardiovascular disease (CVD) factors.[32] For that reason, women who go into early menopause need to pay special attention to their lifestyle choices and habits, and to be open to the possibility of taking estrogen. For them, the estrogen window opens earlier than the standard age of menopause—at the time that they go through early menopause.

Autopsy studies have shown that women who go through early surgical menopause are more likely to have CVD.[33] We also learned from the Framingham study that women who go into early menopause either surgically or naturally are more likely to develop CVD than age-matched premenopausal women.[34] And another large study, the Nurses' Health Study, showed a higher risk of CVD in women who had their ovaries removed and who did not receive HT. Women who had their ovaries removed before age 35 had more than seven times greater risk of heart attack.[35] If women had hysterectomies before menopause but their ovaries were not removed, the risk of heart attack increased by 50 percent. This is because hysterectomy leads to menopause an average of 5 years earlier. In women who had a hysterectomy and ovaries removed, the increased risk of heart attack was even higher. Taking estrogen prevented these increased risks.[36]

Estrogen and Age

The time since menopause, either natural or surgical, is the key to understanding the impact of estrogen on your heart and your estrogen window.[37] We've learned a lot about this from studies of women's arteries.[38] Women who are 35 years old have virtually no plaque in their arteries. Instead they have precursors to plaque called fatty streaks and only very small amounts of actual plaque in their coronary arteries. It's not until perimenopause between the ages of 40 and 50 that plaque becomes present, and after 50 there is a steep increase.[39] The rapid and steady increase in the years leading up to and just beyond menopause is a major reason why women over age 65 have so many heart complications. As mentioned, women have 10 times the number of estrogen receptors on their coronary arteries as men because of the higher amounts of estrogen that women produce. After menopause, when estrogen levels decline, the number of estrogen receptors in women declines and their arteries begin to close—unless they take estrogen during their estrogen window.

The lower estrogen levels deprive the arteries of the positive direct effects of estrogen and as a result, the coronary arteries don't function as well, don't allow blood to flow as well, and slowly become less effective. By 5 to 8 years after menopause the walls of the coronary and carotid arteries that take blood to the brain thicken at the same time that total cholesterol levels and LDL cholesterol levels are rising and adding even more risk to the heart.[40, 41] In women who go through early menopause and do not receive estrogen, it takes about 15 years for all these changes to occur.[42] It's easy to see how all this is a perfect storm for heart disease in women who do not receive estrogen, particularly if they go through early menopause. One of the reasons that women who were originally given estrogen plus progestin women showed an increase in heart attacks and strokes is because HT was given between the ages of 60 and 79, when plaque formation would already have occurred. We now know that when women who already have plaque in their arteries start to take estrogen, it appears to loosen the plaque and increase the risk of complications.[43] These outcomes were from the first WHI study, in which the HT used was Prempro. In the large Finnish study mentioned earlier, the estrogen used was 1 to 2 milligrams of estradiol and the progestin used was largely norethisterone acetate.[44] In that study, women who started HT after the age of 60 did not have an increased risk of heart attack or stroke. That may be due to differences in the lifestyle or genetics of the women, or it may mean that if women do miss their estrogen window and want to begin estrogen, the best choice is estradiol instead of a conjugated estrogen.

The Timing of Hormone Therapy

In the Nurses' Health Study, the 70,533 postmenopausal nurse-participants were between the ages of 30 and 55 when they enrolled, and approximately 80 percent of them began HT within 2 years of the beginning of menopause.[45] The study found that postmenopausal women without a previous history of CVD who started HT close to the time of menopause decreased their risk of future CVD, whereas the few who started their HT 10-plus years after menopause were not protected.[46, 47] In 1998 the Heart and Estrogen/Progestin Replacement Study (HERS), a 4-year trial under the aegis of the National Heart, Lung, and Blood Institute, was undertaken to prove the beneficial cardioprotective effects of an EPT combination therapy.

The average age of the women enrolled was 67, and most began estrogen 10 years after beginning menopause. The study concluded the hormones not only didn't afford the expected protection from heart disease, but they also raised the risk of blood clots in the legs and lungs. On the face of it, this would seem damning. The study design was flawed, however, because the women recruited were already ill with heart disease; 60 percent of the 2,763 participants were lifelong smokers, a known risk factor for heart disease; and the average age of the recruited women was 67, long past both menopause and the estrogen window. The conclusions didn't address the question of estrogen's risk for heart disease in healthy younger women who were at the onset of menopause.

We've talked a lot about the 2002 estrogen and progestin WHI study. There are still a few things to point out in the context of patient selection. The study was supposed to be of healthy women. Now let's look at the reality.

Only 10 percent of the participants were 50 to 54 years old, and 20 percent were between 54 and 59. The rest were 60 to 79. Of the women who received estrogen plus progestin, 36 percent had high blood pressure, 13 percent were being treated for high cholesterol, 4.4 percent were being treated for diabetes, and 10.5 percent currently smoked. In addition, more than two-thirds of the women were either overweight or obese. Given what we've discussed, it's easy to see that many of these women were already at an increased risk of heart attack and stroke.

In an experimental study, when the ovaries of monkeys were removed, the monkeys were fed the equivalent of a high-saturated-fat diet that many Americans eat and immediately given either oral estrogen or a placebo.[48] The size of the plaque in the coronary arteries of those monkeys given estrogen reduced by 70 percent without any change in diet. If the estrogen was delayed slightly after the unhealthy diet was begun, the amount of coronary plaque was reduced by only 50 percent. If the estrogen was delayed for 2 years after the ovaries were removed and an unhealthy diet begun, which is the equivalent of 6 years in humans, there was no protection for the coronary arteries.[49] Similar studies have been done in other animal models with the same results.[50] The reason the estrogen window is so important for your heart is that if the estrogen is begun before significant plaque forms because of lack of estrogen, the potential to protect your heart is at its greatest.

Two more WHI studies came out in 2004[51] and 2011[52] with much less fanfare. They reported that women with a hysterectomy who took estrogen only (ET) were at *less* risk of dying than women who took a placebo; 13 less women per 10,000 died, mostly because of heart disease. In these studies the women were largely 50 to 59 years old, and they began estrogen shortly after the beginning of menopause.

In yet another report[53] of 71,237 postmenopausal women aged 36 to 59, those who only took estrogen had a 46 percent lower risk of dying of

Lifestyle Factors to Avoid Heart Disease

Whether you choose to take estrogen or not, maintaining a healthy lifestyle will improve your chances of avoiding the number-one cause of death in women—heart disease. The nutritional and lifestyle guidelines for preventing heart disease are often the same as those recommended for preventing breast cancer.

- Stop smoking: Smokers have two to six times the risk of heart attack as nonsmokers. The good news is that as soon as you stop smoking, your risk of a heart attack drops rapidly.

- Exercise: It's never too late to start. Walking briskly for 20 to 30 minutes and lifting light weights two to three times per week will help you lose weight and lower your blood pressure, blood glucose, and cholesterol.

- Reduce stress: While there's no proven link between immediate stress and heart disease, chronic stress does cause the adrenal glands to secrete large amounts of the hormone adrenaline, causing your blood pressure to rise, your heart to

heart disease. These studies clearly show that if you are a woman under 59 and you take only estrogen, you will greatly lower your risk of heart disease. This is particularly important if you go through early menopause,[54] which puts women at an even greater risk of heart attack.

More Good News

The Kronos Early Estrogen Prevention Study (KEEPS) done by the Kronos Longevity Research Institute with 727 participants asked two questions: "Does initiating HT in recently menopausal women provide significant protection against hardening of the arteries (atherosclerosis), which is the major cause of heart attacks? Is the alternative way of administering the natural estrogen, estradiol, using a skin patch (a method known as transdermal), equally effective or potentially safer than oral estrogen?"

beat faster, and your breathing to increase. Stress can also increase the release of sugar into your bloodstream.

- Eat a healthy diet: I can't stress it enough, but so much of your total health and well-being depends on what you eat and drink. Focus on eating more greens, beans, vegetables, berries, seeds, and nuts and less saturated fat, salt, sugar, packaged foods, and processed foods.

- Watch your weight: Maintaining your ideal body weight lowers heart risk by 35 to 45 percent.

- Maintain mental health: Treating depression and reducing stress can lower risk.

- Consider aspirin: Check with your health-care provider about taking 81 milligrams of aspirin daily, which has been shown to lower the risk of heart disease. Do not take aspirin if you have liver disease or a tendency to bleed or bruise easily.

After a four-year, double-blind, placebo-controlled trial of low-dose oral or transdermal (skin patch) estrogen and monthly progesterone given to healthy women between the ages of 42 to 59 (average age was 42.7 years) within 3 years after menopause, it was determined that "estrogen/progesterone treatment started soon after menopause appears to be safe; relieves many of the symptoms of menopause; and improves mood, bone density, and several markers of cardiovascular risk."

Remember that the WHI study focused on women aged 60 to 79 (average age was 63), an age range when many women have already developed signs of heart disease, such as atherosclerosis. Atherosclerosis refers to the thickening of artery walls because of calcium buildup in the arteries. When calcium builds up, it becomes difficult for oxygenated blood to flow, which may cause heart disease or stroke. Also unlike the WHI study, the KEEPS study purposely screened out women who showed any evidence of "heart disease (including coronary artery calcium scores of 50 or higher), levels of plasma cholesterol or triglycerides that would normally be treated with lipid-lowering drugs, severe obesity, or a heavy smoking habit."

The KEEPS participants were divided into three groups—those taking oral estrogen, those wearing transdermal patches, and those in a control group—and were measured yearly with a noninvasive ultrasound, MRI, or CT scan to determine whether they developed calcium buildup in the carotid artery (the artery in the neck) during the study.

Whether HT was taken orally—particularly at doses of 0.45 milligram or less—or delivered by a transdermal patch, it had absolutely no negative or positive impact on the participants' heart health during the 4-year study. The KEEPS study showed that younger women can safely take HT during their estrogen window without worrying about heart disease. Ancillary aspects of the KEEPS study showed additional benefits for women who took estrogen: better cognition, improved moods and fewer symptoms of depression, increased verbal memory, and increased libido and orgasms. Even more surprising was that these improvements occurred slightly more frequently in women who used a transdermal patch, rather than taking a pill. More research is being done as the study continues to follow these women.

The bottom line: It's not your age but rather how many years since you went through menopause that determines whether estrogen will be protective or harmful. The longer you go without estrogen, the more plaque there will be in your arteries and the greater the risk of heart attack and blood clots. Starting estrogen close to the time of menopause results in fewer deaths from heart disease. How many? In an article in the *American Journal of Public Health*,[55] the authors concluded that between 2002 and 2011, 42,000 to 48,000 postmenopausal women died prematurely because they didn't take ET.

My findings show that women who take estrogen for at least 5 years within their estrogen window benefit from long-term reduced risk of heart disease and heart failure, with no additional risk of blood clots. It's important to remember that these excellent results only happen when women take the hormone for an appropriate length of time and during their estrogen window.

Chapter 6

The Estrogen Fix and Your Brain

When I began writing *The Estrogen Fix*, I knew that many women would be concerned about the effects of estrogen on their breasts. How could they not be? So much has been written and discussed about estrogen, especially since many of the medications for breast cancer have been created to inhibit estrogen production. While understanding estrogen's role on the breasts is important (see Chapter 4), estrogen also has an effect on many organs and functions throughout the entire body, like the heart, bones, skin, vagina, and, as will be discussed in this chapter, the brain. Once you understand the positive effects of estrogen on the brain, you will be more aware of why it's important to take advantage of your estrogen window as soon as it is open.

When you think about it, your brain helps make you the individual woman you are—your wit, your wisdom, your winning ways. Estrogen can play an essential role in protecting your brain from certain illnesses and slowing the aging process if it is taken at the optimal time. As you'll learn, taking estrogen during your estrogen window provides the best benefits for brain health and a major opportunity for an estrogen fix.

The female brain's relationship with estrogen begins almost at conception, leading it to differentiate distinctly from the male brain while in utero. For example, the corpus callosum—the bridge of nerve tissue that connects the right and left sides of the brain—is thicker in female fetuses than in male fetuses. Research shows that, in general, men's brains connect more strongly from front to back and women's brains connect more strongly from left to right.[1] That's why in general, male brains are "wired" for motor skills, while female brains in general are "wired" to be more analytical and intuitive. Estrogen stimulates the parts of a woman's brain that have to do with emotion and cognition, making women naturally more empathetic and compassionate than their male counterparts.

How Estrogen Protects Your Brain

Estrogen affects neurons throughout the brain[2] and functions both to protect and to stimulate nerves. Brain tissue studied in a petri dish showed that estrogen protects neurons from oxidative stress, low blood-flow, low blood sugar, and damage from amyloid protein, which is believed to contribute to Alzheimer's disease.[3] Estrogen has also been shown to stimulate nerves of the brain to grow, repair when damaged, and transmit signals more effectively through increased branching out of the tips of nerves called dendrites.

Estrogen also affects the neural transmitters between brain cells. These are the chemical messengers that allow one brain cell to communicate with its neighboring cells to say, "Pass it down." How we think, move, feel, and behave—everything the brain controls—depends on the nerves of the brain rapidly communicating with each other to send a message to its destination: pull back our hand from a hot stove, cry when we are sad, put one foot in front of the other to walk or run, analyze a problem, and so forth. And the brain's nerve cells, called axons, communicate by either sending electrical impulses between two nerve cells or by sending a chemical neurotransmitter, such as serotonin, dopamine, or norepinephrine,[4] which is produced in the end of the nerve cells and released into a very small space between itself and the nerve it is trying to communicate with. Estrogen increases the amounts of these transmitters and the speed at which they are released, reabsorbed, or inactivated, all of which have a huge impact on mood. In other words, estrogen helps determine how quickly and efficiently our brains can do its job.

Estrogen also affects the brain's blood supply. Brains need a lot of bloodflow to function at their best. In fact, the brain gets about 15 percent of the bloodflow from the heart[5] in order to meet its oxygen and fuel requirements.[6] Through a complex series of biochemical interactions, estrogen causes the release of nitric oxide in the blood, which causes blood vessels to expand. That, in turn, increases the amount of blood to the brain, which keeps brain tissues well oxygenated and healthy. When a woman is young and is producing lots of estrogen in her body, in addition to all its other jobs, that estrogen is keeping her brain optimally healthy and supplied with a rich, nourishing flow of oxygen. These are all the positive things estrogen can continue to do if a woman takes ET during her estrogen window.

After menopause, especially after early menopause, lowered estrogen levels translate into a lower and less-oxygen-rich blood supply to the brain, and as you can imagine, this can have some pretty serious side effects, including an increased risk of Alzheimer's disease. Yet you can create an estrogen fix and reduce this risk back to normal by taking supplemental estrogen during your estrogen window.

The importance of estrogen on blood vessels has been studied using Doppler ultrasound[7] to determine estrogen's impact on the brain. Menopausal women who did not take estrogen had less bloodflow in their carotid and cerebral arteries than premenopausal women with normal estrogen levels. The further the women were beyond menopause, the lower their brain bloodflow. In another study of bloodflow to the brain, menopausal women had Doppler ultrasound studies of their carotid arteries before and after starting hormone therapy. By the second month of treatment, women taking hormone therapy had significantly improved bloodflow over the entire 52 weeks of the study.[8]

Throughout the body, estrogen also works like an anti-inflammatory to protect the walls of the arteries from developing plaque. The endothelial cells[9] that line arteries have an internal protective mechanism that keeps them working properly and free of plaque. Disease or conditions like diabetes or obesity create inflammation in the blood vessel walls that leads to more plaque and cardiovascular disease. Substances like cytokines and free radicals contribute to the inflammation and are harmful to the endothelial cells.

Another important estrogen fix is how it works on the walls of blood vessels by protecting them from the damaging effects of cytokines that move immune cells toward sites of inflammation or infection and free radicals,[10] and that reduces the risk of developing plaque inside of arteries. This beneficial effect is so powerful that when estrogen was injected into the arteries of rats' brains[11] just before the injection of a toxic substance, estrogen prevented damage to the blood vessel walls. Similarly, postmenopausal women who were followed for 10 years with MRI were found to have less brain injury[12] caused by poor bloodflow *if* they were taking hormone therapy. The longer they took estrogen, the less damage was noted. Estrogen's protective effects on the brain were also observed in both male and female patients who needed emergency resuscitation,[13] specifically those with traumatic brain injury, shock, and sudden cardiac arrest. Typically, the entire focus of treating patients in such situations is to get the heart to start beating again or to get the person breathing again; the focus has not been on protecting the person's brain. When women and men treated for sudden cardiac arrest were also given an intravenous combination of three things—estrogen, a strong antioxidant, and an anti-inflammatory drug—in order to protect the brain and increase survival, brain cell survival of participants treated with this regimen increased by as much as 65 percent. When doctors gave the same regimen intravenously after traumatic brain injury, they observed similar effects.

In a series of studies performed on middle-aged or older animals, increasing estradiol levels increased nerve growth in the hippocampus, increased the growth of capillaries and oxygen flow to the brain, and increased many aspects of learning and memory. Hormone therapy given to postmenopausal women also improved verbal memory.[14, 15] The size of the hippocampus is a good indicator of brain health. The hippocampus is mainly involved with memory, in particular long-term memory. Several studies have found that postmenopausal women who were either currently taking or who had previously received hormone therapy had a larger hippocampus than women who had never taken hormones.[16]

In another study that evaluated the effects of estrogen on the brain, researchers at the Mayo Clinic[17] found that women who had one or both ovaries removed before menopause had a higher long-term risk of Parkinson's disease and of several related conditions known as parkinsonism compared to women who did not have their ovaries removed. Taking estrogen greatly reduces this risk.[18]

Estrogen's ability to improve bloodflow[19] in the brain and reduce other causes of inflammation may be why it has been found to lower the likelihood of depression, Alzheimer's disease, and certain other conditions of the brain and nervous tissues, such as multiple sclerosis and in some reports, even schizophrenia. The reason bloodflow is so important to the brain is that unlike many other organs, the brain can't use reserve fuel sources or alternative metabolic pathways; it depends entirely on bloodflow for fuel.

One of the reasons that women in the 2002 Women's Health Initiative (WHI) study who took EPT had more strokes and some of the other problems that were reported had to do with the fact that Premarin was paired with Provera. Provera works as an antiestrogen,[20] so the positive actions of estrogen were overcome by negative antiestrogen actions of the potent Provera.

Provera makes blood vessels narrow and constrict, and that makes estrogen receptors less sensitive to estrogen and reduces the amount of nitric oxide, so there is less bloodflow to the heart, brain, and other organs. Medroxyprogesterone acetate, which is the generic name of Provera, is 300 times more potent than bioidentical progesterone and is the single most potent downregulator of estrogen receptors, meaning it greatly reduces estrogen receptors' sensitivity to estrogen. These behaviors of Provera can be put to positive use by prescribing it to treat endometrial cancer. But its long-term use contributed to the increased risk of stroke seen with EPT because it so greatly lowered the benefits of estrogen. Provera may also increase the risk of breast cancer.[21]

Hot Flashes and Your Brain

Hot flashes are one of the most common symptoms of and complaints about menopause. Sure, they are annoying, embarrassing, and disruptive. But do they do something much more sinister? Do frequent hot flashes contribute to aging in the brain? Do they leave the female brain more susceptible to aging? Could hot flashes lead to frequent reductions in bloodflow that in turn damage the brain in the way poor bloodflow to the heart leads to cardiac damage? Could they reduce the number of neurons in the brain, particularly in the hippocampus, setting a woman up for Alzheimer's disease?

Some researchers think hot flashes do all these things, which is another reason why women and their doctors need to know about the estrogen window. In addition, women who have surgical menopause have suicidal thoughts twice as often (10%) as women who go through natural menopause.[22]

Women with low estrogen levels caused by removal of their ovaries were found to have memory impairment due to hot flashes.[23] In a separate study using single proton emission computed tomography (SPECT) scans of healthy menopausal women, hot flashes were associated with reduced cerebral bloodflow,[24] and bloodflow is essential to brain health, as described previously. The regions of the brain affected by hot flashes were the same areas where Alzheimer's disease can be seen on a scan. Once the women participants received ET, the hot flashes stopped and cerebral bloodflow returned to normal.[25]

This is particularly important because the volume of the brain and/or its weight naturally reduces at about 5 percent per decade after age 40,[26] and after age 70, brain volume declines even faster.[27] There are gender differences; men tend to lose volume in their frontal and temporal lobes, whereas women tend to lose volume in their hippocampus and parietal lobes.[28, 29] The natural loss of brain volume combined with not being treated with HT seems to be one of the major contributors to Alzheimer's disease, which is more common in women than in men. Women treated with ET and EPT within their estrogen window have not been found to have the same increased risk of Alzheimer's disease as menopausal women not treated with these hormones. It is interesting that one of the major reasons for men having less Alzheimer's disease is that their brains have more estrogen. That's right; men have higher testosterone levels, and both men's and women's bodies can turn testosterone into estrogen by a process called aromatization. As a result, men over the age of 60 have approximately three times more circulating estradiol than women of the same age.[30] It's the reason why men don't begin to lose brain volume until about a decade after women[31]—at age 60.

All these studies help to explain the work of Stanford University researchers who found that estrogen improves verbal memory in postmenopausal women aged 49 to 68.[32] One of the more interesting parts of this study was that the bioidentical estrogen estradiol resulted in significantly better verbal memory performance compared to women receiving conjugated estrogen, although both types of estrogen have been found to improve both verbal and nonverbal memory[33] when compared to a placebo. During this study, women given estrogen for 21 days showed increased activation of their brains when studied with positron emission tomography (PET) scans. It's easy to imagine that having better verbal and nonverbal memory could have a major positive impact on how women feel about themselves because they feel sharper, less foggy, and better focused, qualities that also impact how they are viewed by their family and friends and how they perform at work. Even using estradiol for only 2 to 4 months has been shown to improve verbal memory in woman younger than 65.[34]

Forgetful? Angry? Sad? Irritable? Moody? Teary? Unfocused?

Do you find yourself crying over little things that never bothered you before? Traffic makes you lean on your horn and curse at other drivers? You find yourself screaming at your spouse that he can move out, prepare his own meals, or go back to Mars or wherever he came from for all you care? Or worse?

If you're going through menopause, chances are good that you've experienced at least some or possibly your own version of these wide-ranging emotions. My patients are often stunned and even frightened by the enormous changes and ranges of their feelings. They tell me, "This just isn't me! I've never behaved like this before in my life!"

Well, it is you, and these ups and downs can and often do take place when your brain is going through menopause. All these emotional surges and dips are initially due to the surges and dips of estrogen that slowly lessen in perimenopause and, eventually, much smaller amounts of estrogen that your body produces during menopause. As menopause nears, ovaries can no longer generate either enough or constant levels of estrogen to keep you and your emotions on an even keel.[35] It's bad enough that *you* notice the emotional and physical roller-coaster ride you're on, but often others do too. "Hey, Mom, why are you snapping at me? I just asked a simple question." "Saw you yawning throughout our client meeting. Were you bored?" "We're out of dog food. Did you forget to pick it up on the way home?"

Sound familiar? If your body isn't producing enough estrogen, then the alternative may be ET or EPT, even if used for a window of time. Many women don't realize that ET and EPT might be a huge help in controlling their emotional challenges. They are more concerned about the potential negative effects they have associated with any form of estrogen.

For many women, as menopause approaches, mood swings and irritability are two of the most notable (and distressing) symptoms. In the past you might have felt anxious or a bit sad during certain days of your monthly cycle, but now, in perimenopause, your emotions are more intense and unpredictable. When you think about it, this makes perfect sense; it is caused by an imbalance of estrogen and other hormones that fluctuate wildly up and down.

Ever feel like your brain is working at a slower speed? A little foggy or just struggling to find the answer to a question? If you are in menopause and not taking estrogen, the speed of your brain's processing ability *is* slower,[36] both in processing answers to questions and in reacting to physical changes in your environment.

For example, Enid, one of my patients, was about to step off the curb to cross the street. She told me, "At some level I knew the curb was there, but somehow I didn't process it as quickly as I once did. Instead, I fell and broke my wrist. What a weird experience." Like that of many menopausal women who don't take estrogen, Enid's brain couldn't relay the

BECAUSE Amanda had a 15-year smoking history, perimenopause showed signs of onset (in her case skipping periods) in her early forties. Her physician measured hormonal levels, and they had begun to drop. He encouraged her to think about ET when her levels further declined.

"I put making the decision on the back burner. I was focused on performing well in a new executive position that required a high degree of multitasking and detailed organization. It was not until my manager called me into a private meeting and pointed out slip-ups that I fully realized how much I was struggling with staying focused. Could this be part of menopause?

"I started the recommended dose of Climara using a patch, and my functioning returned almost immediately.

"Years later, my younger sister was diagnosed with breast cancer about the same time the big study on hormones reported dangerous outcomes. I did not want to go off, fearing the return of symptoms. Encouraged by my husband and my doctor to at least try reducing the dose gradually, I relented.

"As a result, I became overwhelmingly sad with frequent bouts of tears and anxiety. We all agreed I should take ET, but at a slightly lower dosage than the original amount and a commitment to be followed closely with mammograms, ultrasounds, and breast checks between annual exams.

"Again, my symptoms disappeared. At age 72, my doctor says I am the oldest woman in his practice and of longest duration to be on ET."

information about the curb to her body as quickly as it should have. Episodes like Enid's are one of the reasons that menopausal women have three times the number of falls as men of a comparable age.[37] Taking estrogen decreased the risk of falling by up to 60 percent over a group of women who didn't take it,[38] according to one study.

Falls are the leading cause of both fatal and nonfatal injuries among aging adults.[39] Combine this with lower estrogen levels and its contribution to osteoporosis and you begin to understand why the benefits of estrogen on both balance and reaction time in the brain are so important.

Most women experience at least some menopause-related moodiness, brain fog, anxiety, and sadness, but they usually are not incapacitated by them. That may not be the case for women who in the past have had disruptive PMS, postpartum depression, or clinical depression;[40] they are at a much greater risk of clinical depression and other mood disorders as menopause approaches. The widely fluctuating and steadily lowering estrogen levels found in menopause often tip them into a mental health challenge. This can be particularly challenging for menstruating women who have both of their ovaries removed and are thrown suddenly into early menopause.[41] Keep in mind that while more than half of all hysterectomies are performed on women aged 45 years or younger, one in nine women between the ages of 35 and 45 have undergone a hysterectomy,[42] and 40 percent of them have had both their ovaries removed at the same time, resulting in an abrupt loss of estrogen and the sudden onset of menopause.[43] When this happens, not only are estrogen levels sent plummeting at an early time, but testosterone levels are also reduced by 40 percent to 50 percent and never go up again, even after these women are well into their sixties.[44] Even if one or both ovaries remain, a hysterectomy may result in the end of ovarian estrogen production—and the beginning of menopause—earlier than usual (by an average of 2 to 3 years).[45, 46] Women who enter menopause in their twenties and thirties, either before natural menopause or because of surgical removal of their ovaries, are at even greater risk of conditions such as heart disease, Alzheimer's disease, mood swings, and Parkinson's disease.

For these women, knowing about their estrogen window is essential to achieving an estrogen fix. Women with premature menopause also have been reported to have more anxiety, depression, somatization (experiencing psychological distress in the form of physical symptoms), sensitivity, hostility, and psychological distress than women who go through menopause closer to the age of natural menopause.[47] So here is the key message: If your ovaries are removed or if for any reason you go into menopause early, you will have entered your estrogen window at an earlier age and to maximally benefit from estrogen, you need to begin it earlier, at the time of early menopause. This concept is reinforced by a study on more than 52,000 women who had surgery for hysterectomy and/or removal of both their ovaries and fallopian tubes for nonmalignant reasons. The investigators followed the women for 22 years and found a 20 percent increased risk of death, mostly due to cardiovascular heart disease, among women who had both tubes and ovaries removed by age 35.[48] The risk of death lowered at 5-year increments in older women who had surgery (i.e., 40, 45, and 50 years). Taking hormone therapy until at least the age of 50 greatly lowered the risk of early death.

Some researchers believe that women who enter premature menopause naturally, not surgically, are demonstrating one component of the entire body aging early. Despite this fact, a recent survey found that one-third of ob-gyns continue to recommend removal of both ovaries in women younger than 51 at the time of hysterectomy in those who are only at average risk of ovarian cancer. These percentages were independent of age, gender of the doctor, or geographic region.[49] If you have a hysterectomy before menopause, have a clear and thoughtful discussion with your doctor about the risks and benefits of keeping your ovaries, especially if you don't have a family history of breast or ovarian cancer, or about waiting as long as reasonably possible if you do.

But estrogen performs an even larger and far more important job in women's brains. After early menopause, lowered estrogen levels translate into a lower and less-oxygen-rich blood supply to the brain that can increase a woman's risk of Alzheimer's disease by 70 percent. Yet taking supplemental estrogen from the time of early menopause until the time of natural menopause can remove this increased risk.

When I first learned this fact during the course of my studies, the increased risk was so large and the beneficial effect of taking supplemental estrogen was so dramatic that I went back just to make sure I had the numbers straight. Women who have early menopause (before age 48) and who do not take estrogen increase their risk of Alzheimer's disease by up to 70 percent—a percentage that is completely reversed by taking estrogen from the time of early menopause until *at least* age 51, the average age of natural menopause.[50]

The strength of the research showing estrogen is beneficial in preventing Alzheimer's is pointed out in a 2015 article in the *Journal of Neurology, Neurosurgery and Psychiatry*.[51] In that article the authors reviewed 16,906 articles on this topic and found that four medications were proven to lower the risk of Alzheimer's disease. Estrogen was first, followed by statins, antihypertensive medications, and nonsteroidal anti-inflammatory drugs.

Menopause and Mental Health

A little brain fog and moodiness is common for many menopausal women. For some, however, menopause puts them at an increased risk of more challenging mental health issues. In fact, some of my patients share with me that they feel like they are "losing their minds." It's important to recognize if you might be at increased risk of depression. Depression is sometimes described as feeling sad, blue, unhappy, miserable, or down in the dumps. But for some women with a history of severe clinical depression or postpartum depression, the transition into menopause can cause thoughts of harming themselves. If any of those feelings surface for you, tell your health-care provider; estrogen may be your answer, but if not,

ELLEN contacted me after she heard me speak about the estrogen window at a conference. As far as her symptoms went, she had suffered through hot flashes and was resigned to just living with them. Cognitive protection—reasoning, memory, and recognition—was what she was most interested in maintaining. Sadly, neither her gynecologist nor her internist felt the cognitive protection offered by ET had yet been proven. But Ellen was really worried. Her mother died in her late seventies with dementia—and Ellen's age, 44, at the onset of menopause after having her uterus and ovaries removed led her to believe she should take estrogen. She would turn 47 within the month and wanted to know if it was too late for her to take ET. Although her estrogen window had been open for several years and her benefits versus risks options were shifting, Ellen had no specific health issues to prevent her from taking ET at her age. I suggested that Ellen tell her doctor about our conversation so she could begin ET as soon as possible.

estrogen plus antidepressants or other treatments can prove lifesaving.

Women who are depressed before menopause, who have had premenstrual or postpartum depression or sexual dysfunction, who are physically inactive, or who have a lot of hot flashes are at more risk of depression as they enter menopause. But women who have not been dealing with any of these issues before they enter perimenopause will overwhelmingly transition into menopause without experiencing severe problems. Still, up to 23 percent of women do report some mood changes, primarily during perimenopause. In fact, in the Harvard Study of Moods and Cycles,[52] premenopausal women with no lifetime history of major depression who entered perimenopause were twice as likely to develop significant depressive symptoms as women who remained premenopausal, and women with hot flashes were at even greater risk. That study also found that women who entered the menopausal transition and who were taking some type of hormonal therapy to reduce their menopausal symptoms or to regulate their cycles did have about the same percentage likelihood of feeling sad or experiencing other depressive symptoms, but they had a decreased risk of developing clinical depression compared with women who did not take any type of hormone therapy.

Part of this has to do with gender differences between men's and women's perception of emotions. Dr. Mark George, while working at the National Institute of Mental Health, performed PET scans[53] on both male and female subjects while asking them to conjure up their saddest memory. PET scans map the flow of blood within the areas of the brain that are active during a given time. To his surprise, the total area of women's brains that was active during memories of strong emotion was eight times larger than the area of men's brains. This may be one of the reasons why women are twice as susceptible to depression as men. There are other differences too. According to scientists at McGill University, serotonin production is 53 percent higher in men's brains than in women's. Serotonin is a brain chemical that is believed to be lower in people who suffer from depression and is the hormone that drugs like Celexa, Paxil, Prozac, and Zoloft, categorized as selective serotonin reuptake inhibitors, known as SSRIs, increase in the brain. One in four women and one in ten men in America will require treatment for depression at some point. If you are being treated with an SSRI, also known as an antidepressant, know that they are associated with loss of bone mass and a higher risk of bone fracture in middle-aged women.[54] So if you're taking one of these medications, talk with your doctor about taking calcium and vitamin D, and about getting regular bone density tests to make sure you aren't developing osteoporosis.

The association between menopause and depression was so high that many women in and around menopause were traditionally prescribed antidepressants. It was observed clinically that SSRIs helped some of those women have fewer hot flashes and night sweats. As a result, SSRIs began to be prescribed off-label (not for the drugs' original intended use) for hot flashes. Brisdelle, an FDA-approved, low-dose SSRI, is now the first approved SSRI offered specifically for hot flashes, though the dosage is too low to actually treat depression. (See page 69 for alternative treatments.) Interestingly, this may be a two-way street; researchers have also found that women with a history of depression were more likely to enter perimenopause earlier than women without a history of depression.[55] Another study also ties in to the relationship between estrogen and depression.[56] Fifty women aged 40 to 55 who were perimenopausal and who had clinical depression were treated with either a placebo or a transdermal estradiol patch of 0.1 milligram. Sixty-eight percent of the women who received the estradiol patch had total relief from their symptoms compared with 20 percent in the placebo group. In a separate study by the same authors, 86.6 percent of women who continued to struggle with depression and who did not respond to estrogen alone did get total relief from their symptoms when an antidepressant was added to the estrogen.[57] If you are in perimenopause and feeling blue, talk with your doctor about treatment with estrogen. You'll be well inside your estrogen window and at the best possible time to begin ET or EPT. If you have not had a hysterectomy and require a progestogen, using bioidentical progesterone will quite likely be a better choice than Provera because Provera has been associated with a risk of depression.

DR. PAULINE MAKI is a professor of both psychiatry and psychology at the University of Illinois in Chicago; a leading researcher in the area of women's health, perimenopause, and menopause, especially emotions, mood changes, and mental health; and past president of the North American Menopause Society. I interviewed her about mood changes in women during the perimenopause and menopause stages of their lives.

DR. MACHE SEIBEL: How big of an issue are mood changes in women as they transition into menopause?

DR. PAULINE MAKI: Mood changes are one of the prominent features of menopausal transition. Research studies show that as women transition from the premenopausal period to the perimenopause and then to the postmenopause, they experience changes primarily in depression and anxiety.

Mood issues, particularly depression and anxiety, affect quality of life in women as they transition through the menopause. Their daily lives are often affected by having increased levels of these symptoms even if they're not diagnosed with clinical depression or other mental illness.

MS: What you're saying is that you may not reach the level where you get an ICD-10 code on a medical slip that says you have clinical depression, but you could be really affected in terms of the quality of your life or the way you have to struggle through a day.

PM: That's exactly right. When women meet the clinical criterion for depression, it means that their symptoms have been so severe and so long lasting that the symptoms negatively impact daily functioning for a period of at least 2 weeks. In contrast, just experiencing higher levels of depressive symptoms means that women don't get as much pleasure, for example, out of their daily lives or they're experiencing higher levels of overall sadness or irritability.

Women often complain of moodiness and irritability when they see their gynecologists for symptoms of the menopause. While hot flashes are the most common reason why women seek help from their gynecologists during the menopausal transition, it's worth noting that there's a very high correlation between mood symptoms and hot flashes in women. The North American Menopause Society recommends that women consider looking for a NAMS (North American Menopause Society) Certified Menopause Practitioner—that is, somebody who is actually certified in the practice of menopause medicine. Those experts understand how symptoms of hot flashes and mental health cluster together among some women as they transition through menopause.

MS: If a woman is feeling sad or blue for more than 2 weeks, then it's a good idea for her to see her doctor or health-care provider?

PM: It's absolutely worthwhile to talk to one's doctor about feelings of sadness and anxiety. It's important to know that there's been a shift in our understanding of menopausal transition as a time when women are at risk for mental health issues even in the absence of any prior history of having these issues.

For example, there are now multiple longitudinal studies that follow women for years as they transition from the premenopausal stage to the perimenopausal stage, and then a few studies on to the postmenopausal stage. The findings show that women, as they transition into menopause, are at an increased risk for both increases in depressive symptoms that are still within the normal range, but higher than what they had when premenopausal, and they are also at higher risk for clinical depression.

The scientific community is now accepting the idea that the menopausal transition is a time period in which some women really need to be alert to the risk for mental health issues.

MS: If you're a woman who has had bad PMS in the past, or you're a woman who has suffered from depression, does that put you at more risk as you go into this window of life?

PM: There is evidence to suggest that women with a history of PMS or postpartum depression are particularly at increased risk for mood symptoms as they transition through the menopause, and women with a history of depression also are at increased risk for mood symptoms during the menopausal transition. Even if you haven't had those risk factors, the menopausal transition is a time period in which women do experience an increased risk of those symptoms.

MS: In addition to anxiety and depression, irritability is also very common. Could you address that?

PM: One of the things that troubles women as they transition through menopause is they feel like their responses to situations have changed and that their responses to a highly emotional situation trigger a larger emotional reaction. As a result, they often react more frequently and with greater responsiveness to situations that once may not have bothered them so much when they were premenopausal. This so-called "irritability" is really the cardinal symptom of a lot of the mood disorders that women experience. The moodiness that women report when we look item by

(continued)

item in our databases is characterized by irritability, which is increased reactiveness to normal situations and getting upset.

One analogy that helps women is to understand that the way they're expressing their mood is very similar to what women express during PMS when they're more emotionally reactive. Women are often relieved to know that what they are experiencing is normal.

MS: How can a woman deal with not feeling that great, being a bit more anxious and sad, and on top of that, knowing her fuse is a little bit shorter?

PM: I wish that I could give you answers based on good clinical trials, for example, the use of oral contraceptives or hormone therapy on these mood issues. Unfortunately, some of that research was halted for a while following the Women's Health Initiative (WHI) study, but the good news is that research has begun again. The WHI study scared some women off hormones because they received messages from the media and health-care providers that hormone therapy was unsafe. The evidence from those initial trials actually found some benefits in mood following treatment with either estrogen therapy (ET) or estrogen plus progestogen therapy (EPT).

A caution, however, is that a hormonal treatment is only going to be helpful if the symptoms were triggered by the hormonal changes of perimenopause and menopause. If a woman is well into postmenopause and develops, for example, depression, hormone therapy would not be effective. She would require antidepressants or other forms of treatment for depression other than ET or EPT. That has been clearly demonstrated.

MS: If you have depression and it's not related to your changing hormone levels, you wouldn't use hormones as an antidepressant, for instance, or as a mood equalizer.

PM: That's exactly right. I would say that the first line of treatment for mood symptoms during the menopausal transition is the use of an antidepressant that also helps with anxiety. Many people who specialize specifically in women's mental health treat on the basis of whether or not these mood symptoms are accompanied by changes in hot flashes. So for a woman who is experiencing mood symptoms and hot flashes, experts in women's mental health will frequently give a hormonal treatment for the hot flashes and night sweats, and then, if needed, they will add an SSRI antidepressant. Other medical practitioners will do the opposite. They'll start with SSRI and then they'll add the hormones.

We also need to be mindful of women who prefer alternative and complementary treatments. For example, there are trials that show improvements in the mental health of women who are transitioning into menopause and who do yoga. There are improvements in mental health in women who tried mindfulness-based stress reduction or hypnotic relaxation therapy as an intervention for hot flashes. Even if these approaches aren't helpful in terms of reducing the frequency of hot flashes, they can provide real benefits to mental health.

Exercise has also been shown to help mild to moderate depression, which is another reason to incorporate healthy behaviors into our daily lives by doing very simple things like parking farther away from the grocery store and taking the stairs rather than an elevator.

MS: A woman who takes an antidepressant may find herself feeling better mentally, but has a lower libido and is less sexually aroused. Do you have any advice?

PM: A recent study showed that women who engaged in vigorous activity for about 30 minutes right before they engaged in sexual activity had a better sexual outcome as a result of it. Women also may want to take a drug holiday in consultation with their doctor. For example, if she knows she is going on a romantic trip somewhere, then she should consult with her doctor about whether or not she could go off her antidepressant for a few days so she feels more romantic while on vacation.

Estrogen and Depression

While it's normal for everyone to feel sad or down every so often, true, ongoing clinical depression is really debilitating and challenging for those who suffer from it. It also impacts their families, friends, and coworkers. There are different kinds of depression, ranging from temporary atypical to postpartum to bipolar disorder. Even though depression has been mentioned earlier, it's such an important topic in today's world that it's worth talking more about it. Depression is about twice as common in women as it is in men, with estrogen, once again, playing a role.

Estrogen is involved in the production of endorphins, the brain's so-called feel-good chemicals, and is tied to increasing levels of serotonin as well as the number of serotonin receptors in the brain. Deficits in serotonin, a chemical created by the human body that works as a neurotransmitter and plays a role in regulating mood, are linked to depression. That's why so many antidepressants, or SSRIs (selective serotonin reuptake inhibitors), work to increase the amount of serotonin available in the brain. Some evidence also suggests that estrogen may even help protect nerves from damage by oxidative stress, an imbalance between the production of free radicals and the body's ability to counteract their harmful effects. Estrogen also increases the concentration of other neurotransmitters in addition to serotonin, such as dopamine and norepinephrine, all of which affect mood and other brain functions.

Although serotonin plays a major role in mental health, it turns out that only 5 percent of serotonin is produced in the brain.[58] Since serotonin does not cross the blood-brain barrier, the serotonin that is active in the brain must be made in the brain. As discussed, the correct amount of serotonin is involved in maintaining a relaxed and positive feeling and in preventing depression and anxiety as well as influencing obsessive-compulsive disorder.

Most of the other 95 percent of serotonin in the body is produced in the intestinal tract, where it can influence the motility of your bowels (how quickly or slowly food moves through your digestive system) and how sensitive your intestines are to pain and fullness.[59, 60] And inflammation in your intestines can influence serotonin in your brain.[61] While all this is still the subject of research, serotonin can be found in lymphatic tissues,[62] and your immune system can change serotonin signals in the central nervous system. This may be the reason that a leaky, inflamed gut can have a major impact on mood.[63]

But here is a really interesting point: Your intestinal bacteria may play an important role in how your body handles estrogen.[64] The more diverse the gut bacteria population of a woman is, the more efficiently she may be able to break down estrogen. In fact, the composition and diversity of the intestinal bacteria were found to be associated with patterns of estrogen metabolism that are predictive of breast cancer risk in postmenopausal women.[65] This study suggested that women whose gut bacteria are more able to efficiently process estrogen may have a lower risk of breast cancer. This study of 60 postmenopausal women between the ages of 55 to 70 is yet another example of estrogen's complex relationship with the brain and gut.

I mentioned earlier that estrogen influences bloodflow to the brain by acting as an anti-inflammatory agent in the walls of blood vessels, protecting them from damage by cytokines and free radicals and impeding plaque formation. It may be that cytokines and their associated inflammation are a common mechanism through which estrogen imparts many of its effects on the brain. For instance, lower levels of estrogen increase the likelihood of depression and postpartum depression. In summary, cytokines are small proteins that allow cells to send signals and thereby increase inflammation. Estrogen lowers their impact and in doing so, lessens their potential negative impact on the brain.

In my practice, I have observed that as menopause approaches, mood swings and irritability are two of the most notable (and distressing) symptoms reported by women. As a menstruating woman from puberty and on, you might have felt anxious or a bit sad from time to time during your monthly cycle, but in perimenopause and menopause, your emotions are more intense and less predictable. This is caused by an imbalance of estrogen and other hormones that fluctuate wildly up and down. The emotional impact of perimenopause is in some ways similar to an extended case of PMS: Hormone imbalance and fluctuations affect the brain with mood imbalance and fluctuations.

If you think about it, it makes sense that some women's brains will be more susceptible to hormonal changes than others. That is why women who have a history of postpartum depression, mild depression, and premenstrual dysphoric depression (a form of PMS) at the beginning of a period are more susceptible to the impact of less estrogen on their brains and more at risk for major depressive disorder as they journey into menopause. Also, women with a history of obsessive-compulsive disorder, panic attacks, anxiety disorder, and other mental health conditions often find that as they enter menopause, their moods become much more difficult to control and their antidepressants or antianxiety medications appear to be much less effective. If you are seeing a psychiatrist for one of these conditions, to get the best

Symptoms of Clinical Depression

According to the American Psychiatric Association, for a diagnosis of depression, at least five of these symptoms must last at least 2 weeks, and at least one of the symptoms must be either (1) depressed mood or (2) loss of interest or pleasure:

- Feeling sad or having a depressed mood

- Loss of interest or pleasure in activities once enjoyed

- Changes in appetite—weight loss or gain unrelated to dieting

- Trouble sleeping or sleeping too much

- Loss of energy or increased fatigue

- Increase in restless activity (e.g., hand-wringing or pacing) or slowed movements and speech

- Feeling worthless or guilty

- Difficulty thinking, concentrating, or making decisions

- Thoughts of death or suicide

results work with your mental health professional and your hormone expert as a team to best help you during menopause. Estrogen may prove very helpful during the transition into menopause, and taking it early in your estrogen window will likely provide you with the smoothest transition.

It's important to find out if your feelings and symptoms of menopause are due to fluctuating estrogen levels, or if something is causing a deeper clinical depression called major depressive disorder. Changing estrogen levels often cause changes in thyroid hormone levels (more estrogen lowers active thyroid levels and vice versa), a cause of depression that can be easily checked for and treated. That's why it is a good idea to check your thyroid levels or thyroid medication dosage when estrogen levels or dosages change. What you are feeling may be due to the hormonal fluctuations of menopause or the unmasking of a deeper clinical depression. Either way, you can be helped in many ways.

Despite the myths and stories of "the middle-aged woman" suddenly becoming depressed or a shrew, the truth is quite the contrary. Sure, there are mood swings, and perimenopausal women often describe PMS-type symptoms. Some women are more sensitive to the effects of estrogen loss on their brains than others. If a woman wasn't depressed before or during perimenopause, it's much less likely that she'll become significantly depressed during menopause.

Depression and mood swings can also be due to diet and hypoglycemia, or low blood sugar. Thyroid disease is also more common in women than in men and is affected by changing estrogen levels, diet, and exercise. Some researchers associate depression with low levels of certain vitamins such as vitamin D,[66] folate, B_{12}, and B_6.[67] A blood test can detect an over- or underactive thyroid and blood sugar and vitamin levels. Both hypoglycemia and thyroid disease can have a major effect on mood and can be treated.

Estrogen and Alzheimer's Disease

Alzheimer's disease is now the sixth leading cause of death in the United States and affects 20 percent more women than men. Countless articles,

DURING Jessica's forty-ninth year, she noticed that she was often more emotional than in the past. She was still having menstrual cycles, but they were much lighter and less frequent than they had been. For the first time, sad movies had her reaching for a box of tissues. Driving in traffic had caused her anger to flare up, so she frequently shared the middle finger of her left hand with other motorists. Jessica felt she was getting a bit out of control and setting a bad example for her teenage daughter. After we talked, Jessica decided to take a bioidentical progesterone in the second half of her cycle to balance her hormone levels. She also signed up for a free meditation app on her smartphone and began yoga classes. In follow-up a few months later, Jessica was still aware of her mood swings but didn't feel the need to act out on them. As her menstrual cycles became further apart, Jessica transitioned to a low-dose estrogen patch in addition to her progesterone to provide her with all the benefits of EPT.

studies, books, TV shows, and movies have been written about dealing with the financial, physical, and emotional costs of Alzheimer's disease and other types of dementia that take enormous tolls on families. Because people are living far longer than they did just 50 years ago, everyone has either been directly affected or knows someone dealing with a relative or friend suffering from the disease. The movie *Still Alice* clearly highlighted the challenges this brings for individuals, families, and friends. Several things make Alzheimer's difficult to deal with—the causes are largely unknown, the disease creeps up quietly, a person can have the disease for many years, and there is no cure. While most people are aware of the disease's mental symptoms, such as memory loss, poor reasoning, and inability to complete tasks, it's usually dehydration, inability to swallow, pneumonia, and/or hip fractures—which lead to other conditions—that ultimately cause death.

There is good news, especially when it comes to Alzheimer's, estrogen, and your estrogen window. Estrogen, which acts like a salve for the brain, has been shown to protect isolated neurons in vitro from oxidative stress, ischemic injury, hypoglycemic injury, and damage by amyloid protein,[68] which is implicated in the pathway to Alzheimer's disease. Estrogen also helps to repair nerves and improve bloodflow to the brain. By 2 months after starting estrogen, ultrasound found that the blood vessels in the brain were showing much more blood passing through the arteries. All these findings are helpful antidotes to aging in the brain. I mentioned earlier in this chapter, but it bears repeating, that in a 2015 review of over 16,000 studies, only four medications were consistently found to lower the risk of Alzheimer's disease; estrogen was rated as number one followed by statins, antihypertensive medications, and non-steroidal anti-inflammatory drugs.[69] The study also mentioned folate, vitamin E/C, and coffee as protective factors of Alzheimer's disease. Depression and current smoking were found to increase the risk.

Hot flashes offer a well-hidden clue about the importance of bloodflow in the brain. This is particularly important because most of the time hot flashes are considered just a nuisance. But hot flashes hide a secret: They cause memory impairment. And one estrogen fix is it reduces hot flashes. Here's another seemingly unrelated clue to the impact of estrogen on women's brain health: In one study,[70] women who had the lowest bone density indicative of lower estrogen also had the worst dementia. All this information suggests that many of the impacts

FIFTY-FIVE-YEAR-OLD Teri had a hysterectomy for abnormal bleeding when she was 52. Over the past few years, she told me she had started to feel increasingly unhappy and more recently, depressed. She had experienced depression years earlier, after her daughter was born, but it went away after 6 months. Hot flashes and heart palpitations became increasingly bothersome.

Teri wanted to discuss hormone therapy but was concerned about the risks. I explained to her that because she had had a hysterectomy and was well within her estrogen window, she was a prime candidate for estrogen-only hormone therapy. Her risks for breast cancer and heart disease would, in fact, decrease on this regimen. Just 1 month after starting estrogen therapy, Teri reported that her mood had improved and the hot flashes were almost entirely gone.

of estrogen we see in one organ of the body are just one representation of how lower estrogen levels can affect other organs of the body.

And when it comes to estrogen and Alzheimer's, it's not only whether or not you take estrogen; it's when you take it that matters. A study found that women who took estrogen within 5 years of menopause (a finding that dovetails neatly with *The Estrogen Fix*) had a 30 percent lower risk of developing Alzheimer's. On the other hand, women who waited and took estrogen at age 65 or later, once their estrogen window had passed, had a 70 percent greater risk of developing the disease. So once again, timing really is everything when it comes to estrogen replacement and the long-term health of your brain and cognitive functioning.[71]

Further evidence of estrogen and its impact on the entire body comes from research on telomeres, the tips of chromosomes that look like plastic caps on shoestrings that prevent the ends of chromosomes from coming unraveled. Telomere length is considered one measure of biological aging; the longer they are, the better. It has been shown that the longer a woman produces estrogen during her lifetime, the longer her telomeres will be. Women have consistently longer telomeres than men, and estrogen exposure might help explain this difference.

To determine whether ET or EPT taken during a woman's estrogen window can protect from the damage that comes with time, a study was done to gauge estrogen's impact on the telomeres of women with the APOE-e4 gene allele. People with APOE-e4 have about four times the risk of developing Alzheimer's disease as those without the gene. APOE-e4 is a major genetic risk factor for Alzheimer's disease and an early death. Telomere length can be used as a predictor of how long you will live, how well you will age, and/or the likelihood of developing certain diseases.

Telomeres normally shorten each time a cell divides. But factors such as oxidative stress, inflammation, and major psychological stress (such as being a victim of child abuse) can cause telomeres to shorten at a faster rate, which is evidence of faster aging.[72] The study followed 63 postmenopausal women (the mean age was 57) who had taken hormone therapy since menopause and randomly divided them into two groups. One group continued their hormone therapy and the other discontinued it.

Over the next 2 years, the APOE-e4 carriers who continued hormone therapy consistently had longer telomeres than the women who did not continue taking it. To be clear, the hormone therapy protected against telomere loss in the APOE-e4 group.

The study also had some surprising results for women who were not carriers of the APOE-e4 gene. For them, stopping hormone therapy actually resulted in longer telomeres at the end of the study. The telomeres of the non-APOE-e4 carriers who remained on hormone therapy did not change during the 2-year study period. Hormone therapy was only added protection for the APOE-e4 carrier group. So estrogen wasn't harmful, but it also didn't add any protection for the noncarriers. This suggests that what women know about their genetic makeup will help determine whether they will benefit from taking estrogen. There weren't enough patients to divide them into groups taking only estrogen and those taking estrogen plus progestin, so there is still more to learn. But for women who are APOE-e4 carriers, hormone therapy seems to offer another layer of protection against Alzheimer's disease.

Estrogen and Weight Control

It's no secret that women become more susceptible to a jelly belly with aging, particularly around menopause when estrogen levels are declining. It's one of the most frequent concerns my patients discuss with me. Estrogen affects weight and weight distribution by directly affecting the fat, the ovaries, and the muscles, which are discussed in other sections of this book. Here I want to discuss estrogen's direct impact on the brain and how that affects weight control.

Researchers at the University of Texas Southwestern Medical Center reported in the journal *Cell Metabolism* an intriguing finding as to why. When estrogen receptor alpha (ER-alpha) was deleted from the entire brain of mice, the mice got very fat. They ate more calories and burned fewer calories. When the researchers deleted the ER-alpha receptors from a specific area of the hypothalamus (SF1 neurons), the mice gained weight without eating more. Loss of ER-alpha receptors from another area of the hypothalamus (POMC neurons) had the opposite effect; the animals ate more without gaining weight. These types of studies suggest there may one day be special types of estrogen that target specific parts of the brain to help control weight.[73]

Estrogen and Sleep

A discussion of estrogen and the brain could not be complete without mention of sleep.[74] Sleep problems are one of the most common experiences for women as they enter perimenopause and menopause; they seem to affect every woman who comes to see me. I typically hear complaints like, "Doctor, I used to fall asleep before my head hit the pillow. Now I stare at the ceiling for an hour before I can fall asleep. Then I wake up several times during the night to go to the bathroom or because I'm dripping wet from night sweats. What can I do?"

How common is this? Studies show that insomnia affects between 11.8 percent and 56.6 percent of women in and around menopause. Of course, a lot of things about menopause affect sleep: hot flashes and night sweats, bladder issues, stress, obesity, and age.[75] If the insomnia is chronic and it isn't treated, it can lead to poor quality of life, decreased work productivity, and more trips to the doctor for a wide range of problems. It's also associated with anxiety, depression, aortic disease, and heart disease. Many major physical and mental problems arise from this very common phenomenon associated with decreased estrogen levels when it occurs around the time of menopause and near the time that the estrogen window opens.

As Shakespeare said in *Macbeth* (act 2, scene 2), "innocent sleep, that knits up the raveled sleeve of care." Poor sleep contributes to the anxiety

FORTY-SEVEN-YEAR-OLD Pamela was in the throes of menopause. Hot flashes and mild anxiety made falling asleep a real challenge. Pamela found that after she finally fell asleep, she would wake up a few hours later and be unable to fall back asleep. She was exhausted during the days, making it impossible for her to stay focused at work. She felt distant from her husband because she was so tired; she had no interest in sex. One day while on her way home from work, she feel asleep for a split second at the wheel while driving. That frightening episode caused her to schedule an appointment to see me.

Once we reviewed her blood tests and talked about her symptoms, Pamela began using a low-dosage estrogen patch. Within 2 weeks, she fell asleep without tossing and turning. If she woke up to go to the bathroom or just to turn over, she fell right back to sleep. In a few months, her mood and energy were back up to their former levels, her effectiveness at work improved, and she was again enjoying an intimate relationship with her husband.

and depression that so many women experience as they transition into menopause. Quite interestingly, a recent study found that the timing of hot flashes may contribute to whether or not they cause depression. When hot flashes interfere with falling asleep or cause early awakening, depression is far more likely.[76] While most adults need 7 to 8 hours of sleep per night, the National Sleep Foundation estimates that 46 percent of women aged 40 to 54 and 48 percent of women aged 55 to 64 have issues getting a good night's sleep.

My experience has taught me to ask my patients if they are having trouble sleeping, because they often don't think it's worth mentioning, or they believe that lack of sleep is so common they should just grin and bear it. An additional contribution to poor sleep's impact on women is that during perimenopause and menopause, sleep is not only reduced in quantity but also in quality. While not getting enough sleep is partially caused by low or fluctuating estrogen levels, other problems, such as getting up at night to go to the bathroom, reading electronic devices just before bedtime, restless legs, hot flashes, and sleep apnea explain why perimenopausal and menopausal women are more than twice as likely to use prescription sleep aids than premenopausal women.

Poor sleep is not just about being tired. Not getting enough sleep has a major impact on your health and well-being. Women who sleep too little have decreased memory and increased irritability, and they tend to gain weight. Weight is affected because leptin, the hormone that makes you feel full after eating, is produced during sleep. Less sleep leads to less leptin,[77] which causes hunger and cravings. The hungrier you feel, the more you will eat. Poor sleep also increases stomach production of ghrelin, a hormone responsible for making you feel hungry.

Lack of sleep has also been linked to increased risk of heart disease, high blood pressure, and diabetes. A person is said to have adequate sleep if she can function in an alert state during her desired waking hours. Poor sleep (either too little or poor quality) can lead to poor performance on the job, and this can play a major role in how one is perceived at work. Poor sleep can also cause muscle aches, irritability, poor motivation, and fatigue.

It's hard to sleep through drenching night sweats when your night-clothes and bed linens are repeatedly soaked from perspiration. Getting up frequently to go to the bathroom to urinate is disruptive. Other causes of poor sleep include arthritis pain in joints, obesity, depression, stress, and anxiety. Once again, estrogen, or the lack of it, plays a role in menopausal women not getting enough sleep. Low estrogen levels have been shown to

KITTY, who quit smoking at age 42, went through menopause in her late forties. "What I remember most about that time is that I swear I didn't sleep for 6 months. Hot flashes and night sweats kept me staring at the ceiling all night. I'd finally fall asleep at 5 or 6 in the morning. I was completely unable to focus and pay attention at work. I came in late at least 3 days a week because I just couldn't pull myself out of bed."

Kitty's doctor first recommended over-the-counter remedies, which didn't have any effect. A hormone specialist then prescribed estrogen-only tablets with progesterone to be taken only on certain days.

"Within a month, I was blissfully sleeping through the nights. I took estrogen and progesterone for approximately 12 years. I don't know how I would have managed without it."

shorten rapid eye movement, the deep, satisfying period of sleep your body needs to feel fully rested. As a result, you're just not getting the refreshing sleep your body requires to think and work efficiently. To download a free sleep diary to help you track your sleep so you can discuss your sleep patterns with your doctor, visit FreeSleepInfo.com.

The Estrogen Fix and Women in the Workplace

If you are a woman in or around menopause, you know that at times menopause creates special challenges for work and vice versa. I've listened attentively as hundreds of my patients described awkward moments such as hot flashes during a meeting, brain fog and forgetting to turn in a report, tiredness due to poor sleep that makes them appear uninterested, constantly peeling off layers of clothes and adding them back to control their changing temperature, and embarrassing moments and near misses from too few bathrooms strategically located for women with sensitive bladders. All this can affect a woman's work ability, a term used to describe effectiveness in the workplace.

Women provide essential income for their families[78] and represent over 47 percent of the full- or part-time US labor force. More than 57 percent of women in the United States are working.[79]

In 2014, the percentage of women who participated in the work force by age were:

AGE	% WOMEN WORKING
35–44	74.1%
45–54	73.8%
55–64	58.8%
65 and over	15.1%

U.S. Bureau of Labor Statistics, Current Population Survey, 2014 annual averages, bls.gov/cps/cpsaat03.htm.

As you can see, millions of women are working at age 51, the average age of menopause, and the numbers of working women are on the rise. By 2022, over two million women between the ages of 65 and 74 will be working, representing 31.9 percent of that age group. The benefits of work are more than income. Women who work tend to have higher self-esteem, better health, and less psychological stress.[80, 81]

Since so many of the women in the workplace are in perimenopause, menopause, or postmenopause, it's important to understand the impact it has in the workplace and to realize that things can and should be done to help. In most countries, women have higher rates of sickness absence than men, and older workers have higher rates of sickness absence than younger workers. And several studies show that women aged 45 and older have the highest incidence of sickness absence.[82, 83]

A study performed by Dr. Marije Geukes and colleagues was done to examine the impact of menopausal symptoms on work ability.[84] They studied all female employees aged 44 to 60 at a hospital in the Netherlands and found that menopause had a significant impact on work ability.[85] Work ability is a concept widely used in occupational health that can predict both future impairment and duration of sickness absence. Women in menopause tested as though they were impaired. A separate study discovered that women around the age of 51 were most likely to have declining work ability, and women with severe hot flashes were almost three times more likely to have their work ability impacted than women with mild to moderate hot flashes. Sleep disturbances also play an important role[86] in negatively affecting women in the workplace.

SANDRA YANCEY is founder of eWomenNetwork, a multimillion-dollar enterprise in six countries that helps thousands of women grow their businesses.

Sandra has been named by the International Alliance of Women one of the world's 100 Top Difference Makers and by CNN as an American Hero. The eWomenNetwork Foundation has awarded grants to 101 nonprofit organizations and scholarships to 147 emerging female leaders of tomorrow.

DR. MACHE SEIBEL: Sandra, thank you very much for discussing women, menopause, and work.

SANDRA YANCEY: Oh, Dr. Mache, thank you. I think what's most relevant and important for our conversation is that something happens to women once they hit 40. I know the statistics show that we live a lot longer than 80 today, but generally speaking, at least from a business-career perspective, our careers are only half

(continued)

over at 40. And many of us are mothers. I didn't have my first child until I was 30, my second child when I was 35, so I had them a little bit later than many women. Yet when I hit 40, I found myself thinking about how I wanted my life to be different than it had been. I began to think about reimagining my life.

MS: Did something in particular happen when you turned 40, or did the "Oh, no 4-0" just stare you in the face and you said, "Self, I'm 40. It's time for me to get my act together." What happened?

SY: I had a daughter who was almost 10 and a son half her age, and I just thought to myself, "Gosh!" Brianna was about to enter her preteen years, and she was always a little bit early. I thought to myself, "If I do this right, they're going to be very crystal clear on their purpose and their goals and they're going to fly the nest and they're going to live their own life." And I thought to myself, there's going to be a lot of life left in me.

MS: You were anticipating being an empty nester and rather than wait, you said to yourself, "Where am I, who am I, and what will I be doing?"

SY: Yes, that's indicative of my style. I'm a big planner. A lot of people announce their resolutions on January 1. I announce mine on October 1, and I spend the last quarter of the year preparing for January 1 so that when the doors open and when the ball comes down, I'm off to the races.

MS: I would like to ask you a question if you are open to talking about it, and that has to do with the concept of hormones in the transition toward menopause. One of the things that many women do not realize is the impact that this time of life has on many women in the workplace. What can you tell women about being open to getting their symptoms treated so their symptoms don't make life and work more challenging?

SY: I would say treat yourself as you would treat your child. If you saw your child experiencing a symptom that you knew was not in alignment with how the body should be functioning at its optimum best, would you allow that chronic situation to continue over time?

They would not, of course. It's like getting on a plane. The flight attendant—I don't care what plane you're on—always stands up and says, "Should we go through some turbulence, a little yellow oxygen mask is going to drop out of the ceiling. Put it on your mouth and nose first and start breathing and then assist passengers traveling with you."

We've got to learn to start taking care of ourselves. I had less hot flashes, but I did experience night sweats. What I can tell you was I realized that the interruption in my sleep was impacting my effectiveness at work, and I knew that my body was going through some shifts and some changes and all I wanted to do was learn what I could do to help minimize them in a way that kept me functioning optimally; my sleep, my temperament, and my feelings. All those things that get out of whack when you start to go through menopause.

Going through the change ended up being *the* most wonderful productive time of my life.

MS: You're at your peak. You have all your experience, your wisdom. You're a role model, a mentor, you have a chance to impact your company. But the company can also benefit from your dynamism; it doesn't go so well when a person is tired, foggy, or moody.

SY: Totally. I wouldn't change this time in my life for anything. I can honestly say I've enjoyed every phase just like I enjoyed all the phases of my children, the pluses and the minuses at times, of course.

But this is a very empowering time, particularly because for most of us we're ending the child rearing, to take all of that energy and focus and begin to turn it inward and really take responsibility for taking care of ourselves. For no other reason, I want to be a role model for my own daughter.

That means putting yourself on the list, eating well, exercising, and getting enough sleep. I believe in meditation and reflection, being in gratitude, focusing on the positive. Those are, I think, the ingredients for living not only a healthy life, but living an inspired and inspiring life, and this is a wonderful season.

In another report, Dr. Phil Sarrel of Yale found that two-thirds of women reported that their menopausal symptoms had a moderate to severe effect on their work, and some had to quit work as a result.[87] Dr. Sarrel commented that 95 percent of women who were corporate executives experienced physical symptoms, and 79 percent experienced emotional symptoms related to menopause.[88, 89] The most common symptoms that challenged the women were insomnia, night sweats, and hot flashes. All these can be treated. And at the time the study was performed (2008–2009), 39 percent of women had stopped using HT because of the negative WHI findings. Currently, only about 15 percent of postmenopausal women are using either ET[90] or EPT.

It's easy to see the impact of the WHI study on women in the workplace. Women continue to rise in their impact on all levels of the workforce and continue to constitute a rising percentage of people working. At the same time, women's work ability is being challenged in large part by fear of estrogen, which I'm calling "estrophobia."

Evidence of the impact of the WHI and fear of estrogen can be seen in the changing demographics of women in the workplace. An article in the *New York Times* reported that according to the Bureau of Labor Statistics, although the total number of women in the workplace has continued to grow, the participation rate of a single age group has decreased over the past decade: ages 45 to 54. All other age groups of women have increased in the workplace.[91]

According to the bureau, one million women aged 45 to 54 have dropped out of the workforce during the last decade despite absolute numbers increasing. While we can't say with total certainty that this decline is due to not taking estrogen, the fact that this huge group would mysteriously disappear from the workforce at a time of life when they are most productive is at best puzzling. Those dropping out include bank presidents, head nurses, and self-employed business owners. We know from studies of work ability that the symptoms of menopause make it challenging for women in this age group to handle the demands of work. This translates into 3.5 percent of the 45-to-54-year-old women dropping out of the workforce since 2007 (5 years after the findings of the 2002 WHI were reported). For younger women the rate of decline was about 2 percent, mostly due to taking care of children; for those age 55 and older, there was an increase of 4.2 percent. Part of the reason for this decline in women aged 45 to 54 was attributed to the fact that most employers do not offer flexible schedules for workers caring for elderly family members and their own dependent children and young adults living at home.

According to the *New York Times* article, AARP's Public Policy Institute estimated that women 50 and older who permanently left the workforce to care for a parent lost nearly $325,000 each in wages and benefits.

Why isn't more being done to help women at this time of life, especially in light of all the evidence? Is it just the challenges of work and life that caused one million women to depart the workforce in their prime? Could they have coped better and been better able to continue working if their menopausal symptoms had been treated? A report in the March 2015 issue of the journal *Menopause* reported on their review of the insurance records of half a million women at *Fortune* 500 companies for a diagnosis of hot flashes.[92] Of the approximately 500,000 women, half (250,000) were treated for their hot flashes and the other 250,000 were not. The 250,000 women with hot flashes who were not treated had approximately 1.5 million office visits over the 12 months of the study. This impacted their work ability, effectiveness at work, and productivity and cost the insurance companies hundreds of millions of dollars. All because of hot flashes that were not treated. Had these women fully understood their estrogen window, it is likely that most of them would have considered estrogen or at least an estrogen alternative and been better able to balance work and life. Understanding the estrogen window is absolutely essential for both the women and the businesses in which they work.

Women in their estrogen window are at a time of their careers when they have experience, wisdom, and the potential for impact. They can serve as role models for other women. It is really important that they understand how to best deal with their menopause transition, because when they do, they can remain effective in the workplace, often in leadership positions, and can effect workplace change to help other women and increase organizational awareness. Numbers of bathrooms and distance to them, flexible times for work, and cooling systems that account for hot flashes are just a few of the changes that can be implemented. I talk about these things in my lectures and workshops to women's organizations, businesses, and women's groups. Employee health benefits could be expanded to include programs like the MenopauseBreakthrough.com online program we have developed to guide women either individually or in the workplace through this challenging transition. The whole point is to embrace menopause and increase understanding so the symptoms can be treated, and that can only be done through educational forums.

(continued on page 136)

Lifestyle Changes to Improve Your Sleep

Making some simple changes in your life can help to improve your sleep during perimenopause and menopause.

Estrogen not only improves sleep by reducing night sweats, it also increases REM sleep. For women who prefer not to take a full regimen of estrogen, I suggest a low dose of oral estradiol at bedtime. It lasts in the blood for about 8 hours and acts as a surrogate sleeping pill. Whether you choose to take estrogen or not, the good sleep hygiene suggestions below will help.

- Don't watch the late news. Think of all the negative things typically reported on the evening news: rapes, murders, bombings, financial problems, and other heartaches. This negative input just before bedtime plants a seed of thought, and our brains like to process the last things we think about. It's called dream incubation and is used intentionally by some people to solve problems. For a more restful sleep, wind down at least 2 hours before bedtime—no TV, computers, e-mails, or smartphones. Instead listen to relaxing music, take a relaxing bath, read a relaxing book, or have a relaxing talk with friends. Note the frequent use of the word *relaxing*.

- Use associate activation to connect going to bed with a positive experience. In this process, ideas that have been evoked trigger many other ideas. It's very complex neuroscience, but as an example, you link together two words, like *bed* and *happy*. Your brain starts to involuntarily make a story of this. And in an amazing, virtually immediate sequence of events, your brain takes this nugget of a thought and creates a ripple effect that becomes the story your brain is telling you. Think of positive words or phrases at bedtime to associate your slumber with good things.

- Prime your brain to lower anxiety and sleep better. Nobel Prize laureate Daniel Kahneman describes this process in his book *Thinking Fast and Slow*. He tells of an experiment in which the participants were told they were testing the quality of audio equipment and were instructed to move their heads to check for distortions of sound. Half were instructed to nod their heads up and down, while the other half were directed to shake their heads from side to side. The ones who nodded up and down tended to feel favorable about the editorials they heard; the ones who shook their heads from side to side tended to reject the editorials' hypotheses. Once again, positive actions led to positive behaviors. Engage in things you enjoy doing before bedtime.

• Go to bed at the same time each night, avoid large meals before bedtime, and don't use caffeine, alcohol, or nicotine near bedtime.

• Use a white noise machine or app to block undesirable sounds. These come with all kinds of soothing sounds, from heavy rainfall to a babbling brook that will block out loud neighbors, a snoring partner, or traffic.

• Sleep in a darkened, cool room. Use an eye mask or purchase room-darkening shades. It's easier to fall asleep in a cool, rather than a warm or hot, environment. Creating a true sleep environment will help you fall and stay asleep.

• Exercise is a great and effective antidote for chronic insomnia.[93] Even a single exercise session of moderate-intensity aerobic exercise like walking reduces the time it takes to fall asleep and increases the length of sleep compared to a night not preceded by exercise.[94] However, in the same study, more vigorous aerobic exercise such as running or weight lifting did not improve sleep. As people began to exercise more frequently for 4 to 24 weeks or longer, adults with insomnia fell asleep more quickly, slept slightly longer, and had better sleep quality than before they began exercising.[95, 96]

• Write it down. If you have unresolved issues at work or a problem on your mind, write it down on a pad with a pen kept

(continued)

Just as some companies are friendly to pregnancy, maternity leave, childcare centers, lactation rooms, and flexible work hours, it's time to provide the same attention to the other special times in a woman's life. The benefit would not only be to have happier, healthier, more effective workers, but also to improve productivity for the companies providing this. It's time to realize a major brain drain of women are leaving the workforce at their peak potential, and this could be addressed with education, awareness, and planning. To find out more about our workshops, lectures, and online programs, visit DrMache.com. My hope is that as women become aware of their estrogen window, they will consider estrogen or other treatments so they can be healthier and more effective in all aspects of their life.

As you have read, estrogen plays a major role in your brain. Estrogen improves sleep, bloodflow, and cognition and has a favorable effect on mental health challenges, particularly in perimenopause and menopause. Estrogen fights Alzheimer's disease, inflammation, and brain aging and improves your work ability. And estrogen is most effective if taken during your estrogen window.

Chapter 7

The Estrogen Fix and Your Bones

Most people don't think about their bones much until they break or ache. Unlike our teeth, our bones are buried beneath our skin, muscles, and fat. Like so many other parts of a woman's body, bones have a close relationship with estrogen and the estrogen window.[1]

The bones are where the body stores most of its calcium. As girls develop into young women, they incorporate literally pounds of calcium into their bones to help them grow. The majority of the body's growth is complete and bone density is at its highest by the time a young woman reaches her late teens and early twenties. Medically speaking, bone density refers to the amount of mineral matter per square centimeter of bone. Calcium and magnesium are most essential for bone growth, but vitamins C, D, and K and small amounts of trace minerals, such as copper and zinc, also play important roles. Calcium is necessary for body functions such as muscle and nerve function, blood clotting, and others.

Bone is living tissue. Bone tissue constantly breaks down and rebuilds and repairs itself. Compact bone is the strong, hard outside part of the bone that makes up most of the human skeleton. Cancellous bone is the spongy tissue inside compact bone where red and white blood cells are formed in the marrow.

Calcium is about 1.5 to 2 percent of our body weight. About 98 percent of the approximately 3 pounds of the calcium in our body is in our bones, about 1 percent is in our teeth, and the final 1 percent is in other tissues and in our circulation[2] at a concentration of about 10 mg/mL. When calcium beyond what is taken in from our diet is called on to carry out certain functions, parathyroid hormone increases. This leaches calcium out of the bones, and increases absorption from our intestines, so our bones must absorb more calcium to maintain its effectiveness[3] and to prevent weakening of the bones. Failure to adequately absorb calcium is one cause of bone loss from osteopenia (when bones are not as strong as they should be because of loss of calcium) and osteoporosis (when bones are so weak, they easily fracture). At their simplest level, bones are constantly in a state of remodeling, which is the term used to describe their natural breakdown and repair process. Osteoblast cells build bone; osteoclast cells break bone down. During the years of growth and higher estrogen levels in women, there is more osteoblast activity than osteoclast activity. During most of a woman's adult years, these two cell types stay in balance. In menopause, because estrogen does suppress osteoclasts somewhat, the roles are reversed, and osteoclast activity becomes greater than osteoblast activity as estrogen levels decline. It's also important to mention the role of testosterone, which stimulates osteoblasts.[4, 5] For women who have had a hysterectomy and who are taking estrogen and still losing bone density, adding testosterone can help. Estrogen slows the osteoclasts' breakdown of bone; testosterone increases the action of osteoblasts to build more bone.

The bones contain estrogen receptors, particularly the alpha receptors, which allow estrogen to stimulate them. Estrogen increases the activity and number of osteoblast cells. These cells place calcium into bones to fill in cracks and hairline breaks and help bones grow and stay strong. Lack of estrogen causes more bone to be broken down and removed as calcium enters the bloodstream[6, 7] to participate in the physiology of the body. In essence, the bones are the calcium savings account of the body. The more calcium you store in your bones earlier in life by maintaining a diet rich in calcium, exercising regularly, and not smoking, the stronger your bones and the greater your "calcium savings account" will be as you age.

As women enter perimenopause, menopause, and beyond and estrogen levels become lower, their bones also enter their estrogen window. The estrogen receptors on bone cells[8] that allow estrogen to exert its actions start to decline, and the activity of osteoclasts increases. With lower levels of estrogen, inflammatory cytokines increase (just like they do in the blood vessels) and contribute to faster bone loss.[9] These bone-losing processes that occur naturally with lower estrogen can be reversed with estrogen[10] or with SERMs (selective estrogen receptor modulators) that work by selectively stimulating the estrogen receptors on bones.

Without question, science has established that estrogen is crucial for bone health in women and is an estrogen fix. When estrogen production is reduced in postmenopausal women, their bones slowly develop osteopenia and osteoporosis and become brittle and break more easily. Even in the 2002 WHI study and many others that have followed, ET and EPT have been shown to lower the risk of osteoporosis. And as is true with most other tissues, there is an estrogen window. Early interventions pay great dividends. Research done by Dr. Robert Lindsay helped to fine-tune the estrogen window for bone (see figure below). When the ovaries were removed, causing surgical menopause, and estrogen was replaced immediately, there was no bone loss over the next 12 years. If after removal of both ovaries there was a delay of 3 years before beginning estrogen, those women lost 10 percent of their bone density. But if estrogen was given at that time, the bones were able to regain the lost density. If 6 years passed after removal of both ovaries before estrogen was taken, there was no additional bone loss, but the bones were also unable to regain any of their lost density. So the estrogen window for bones appears to be about 6 years, but it is most effective if estrogen is begun as early as possible after surgical menopause.[11]

Effect of Delay of Onset Estrogen Treatment on Bone Loss

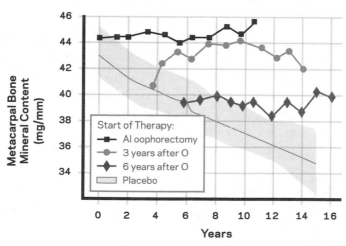

R. Lindsay, D. M. Hart, et al., "Bone Response to Termination of Oestrogen Treatment," *Lancet* 1, no. 8078 (June 24, 1978): 1325-27.

How Cancer Can Lead to Bone Loss

- Some chemotherapy drugs lower the body's calcium levels.

- Pelvic radiation therapy, especially for women over 65

- Cancer can spread (metastasize) to the bone from where the tumor was originally.

- Hormone therapy to suppress estrogen in breast cancer patients

- Steroid treatments such as prednisone pull calcium out of bones.

Osteoporosis, or thinning of the bones, leads to compromised bone strength, which is the most common bone disorder in humans. It affects 28 million Americans, and 80 percent of them are women. About half of Caucasians, Hispanics, and Asians and 38 percent of African Americans have bone loss that can lead to osteoporosis. Potential osteoporosis is one of the most significant threats that can come with menopause. Unless you have a bone density test, you might not even be aware that this silent disease can cause loss of height, a broken hip or other bones, or even death. If you are a woman over 50 who has osteoporosis, your risk of breaking a bone doubles every 7 to 8 years. (By the way, men do get osteoporosis, but usually about a decade later than women when their testosterone levels drop.)

This is important to know because about 300,000 Americans fall and break their hips each year, and 70 percent of them are postmenopausal women. Taking estrogen during your estrogen window lowers that risk by 60 percent.[12] This is one of the places where Provera plays a positive role because it also helps reduce the risk of hip fracture. Although it is not as effective to begin ET after age 60, there is evidence that it can still help prevent further loss of bone, and that may be sufficient to prevent a hip fracture.

Bone loss begins to accelerate a few years before menopause as estrogen production decreases, eventually leveling off about 3 years after menopause.

During this time women annually lose about 2 percent of bone. That can quickly add up, especially if you didn't eat enough calcium-rich foods as a youth, when your bones were developing and growing. During the years around menopause you can lose 10.5 percent of your spine's bone density and 5.3 percent of your femoral neck bone density, where a hip fracture takes place. Women who go through menopause early or who have pelvic radiation or chemotherapy have even lower bone density.[13] A recent follow-up review of the menopausal women in the original WHI studies found that those who went into menopause before age 40 and did not take estrogen were 20 percent more likely to have a bone fracture than women who went into menopause at age 50 or later.[14] After the estrogen window around menopause closes, bone density loss is about 1 to 1.5 percent per year.

Bone Density

When you see an elderly woman (or man, for that matter) who is stooped over, it usually means that she has *osteoporosis,* a progressive bone disease involving decreased bone mass and density due to calcium loss. *Osteopenia,* thinning of the bones, is an early warning sign that precedes osteoporosis. Some loss of bone mass and density is natural as we age, especially in menopausal women, and it can lead to a fractured pelvis or other broken bones. If osteopenia or osteoporosis is diagnosed early, there are treatments.

Some doctors recommend waiting until age 60 to 65 to get a bone density test, but I strongly disagree. By then the horse is out of the gate, and it's too late to take measures to prevent the problem. I tell most of my patients to get a baseline bone density test at age 50 and then have a second one 1 or 2 years later to see if any more bone has been lost in that amount of time. It takes two dots to make a line and see if it is angled up (bone more dense), down (bone loss), or level (no change). If there is bone loss during those 12 to 24 months, then a density test should be done every year. If there is no bone loss, then bone density tests can typically be done every 5 years. Women who at are high risk of osteoporosis (smokers, those with a family history of fractures and osteoporosis, and those who take steroid, thyroid, and other medications that can contribute to bone loss) should have their first bone density test at age 40 and every year after. If bone thinning is found early, it can be treated and bone fractures can be prevented.

Bone Density Test

A bone density test (DEXA, or dual-energy x-ray absorptiometry) is the best way to determine bone density and to show if there is loss. Once the bones have lost a lot of calcium, it is harder to get it to return. Finding bone loss early is the best way to prevent a hip fracture when you are 70 or older. It is a noninvasive, painless x-ray procedure that measures how many grams of calcium and other important minerals are compressed into your bones. The radiation exposure is minimal, about 10 percent of the radiation received in a routine chest x-ray. Measurements of the lower spine, hips, and sometimes the wrist are taken, since those are the bones most likely to break if weak. A bone density test will confirm if you have osteoporosis and can help monitor your treatment.

Tips to Prevent Osteoporosis and Broken Bones

- Get early detection. The sooner you find evidence of bone loss, the quicker you can treat it. A bone density test can determine if bone loss is occurring.

- Eat calcium-rich foods or take calcium and vitamin D_3 supplements. Calcium decreases as we age, so it's important to replace it with calcium-rich foods or supplements. Also, the stomach becomes less acidic with aging and absorbs less calcium. Calcium-rich foods include cheese, fat-free milk, yogurt, and dark green vegetables, or calcium-fortified foods like orange juice. Vitamin D helps your body absorb and retain calcium, as does magnesium. Have your 25-hydroxy vitamin D level checked. Other minerals, such as magnesium, are also involved in building healthy bone, and taking a magnesium supplement daily can be helpful. Here's a tip: Don't take a magnesium supplement at the same time as the calcium supplement, or most of it won't be absorbed. It's also important not to take more than 600 milligrams of calcium at once for the same reasons. Your body can only absorb so much at one time, so take these supplements at least several hours apart. Visit EstrogenFixBook.com for a

A bone density test yields two scores, a T score and a Z score. The T score indicates how much bone density you have compared with a young adult of the same gender with peak bone mass. Here is how to interpret your T score:

T SCORE	INTERPRETATION
Above -1	Normal
-1 to -2.5	Osteopenia
Below -2.5	Osteoporosis

The Z score indicates the amount of bone you have compared to other people in your age group and of the same size and gender. If it is

list of calcium-rich foods and how much calcium they contain.

• Take bisphosphonates: Check with your doctor to see if Fosamax, Boniva, or some other prescription medication that slows the rate of bone loss and may promote new bone growth is appropriate for you.

• Exercise: Weight-bearing physical activity like walking and dancing stimulates the body to make bone-forming cells (osteoblasts) and helps build muscles to keep you strong and stable.

• Maintain a healthy weight: Healthy bones require a healthy diet. Being underweight increases the risk of bone loss and fractures. Being overweight stresses bones, especially the knees and hips.

• Prevent falls: Keep your environment free of things like scatter rugs and clutter that could cause you to trip, fall, and break a bone.

• Have your vision checked annually: Not seeing well is one of the most common reasons that people fall, as when the bathtub edge is higher or the doorknob is farther away than expected.

unusually high or low (less than -2.5 or above +2.5), it may indicate a need for further medical tests.

It's normal to become shorter as we age, and you may not notice it, especially if your bone density test results are normal. Perhaps you've measured 5 feet 5 inches tall since you were 15 years old, but now find that you're 5 feet 3½ inches tall at age 65. As the spine thins from osteoporosis, the vertebrae, or cylinder-shaped bones that line up to form the backbone, can start to compress. It's like an empty tin can that someone squashes. As the vertebrae get squashed, the bone compresses. I've had several patients tell me they don't understand why they are getting shorter, yet their bone density is normal. Their bone density isn't really normal. It just looks normal because compressed thin bone suddenly looks denser. The goal is to find this problem before it gets to this point and treat it so it doesn't happen. Taking estrogen during your estrogen window is one way. Many other treatments are now available as well. For a list of osteoporosis treatments, visit EstrogenFixBook.com.

FRAX

Fracture Risk Assessment Tool (FRAX) is an online tool (shef.ac.uk /FRAX/) to help you estimate your bone fracture risk. The FRAX tool takes into account your bone density T score as well as other factors like your age, height, and weight; smoking history; alcohol consumption; other health conditions such as rheumatoid arthritis; whether or not you take corticosteroid medications; and your family and personal history of fractures. The online tool helps to predict your risk of fracture in the next 10 years. FRAX can help determine whether you would benefit from treatment for osteoporosis.

Calcium and Vitamin D

Calcium and vitamin D are two of the important nutrients our bodies need to maintain strong bones. In addition, calcium is important for the normal function of the heart, muscles, and nerves. You can get some idea of how many functions calcium has when you think of the medications called calcium channel blockers.[15] These medications affect the movement of calcium in the body and are used to treat everything from high blood pressure to chest pain and migraine headaches. Inadequate

WHEN she came to see me, 64-year-old Beverly said that dealing with hot flashes was difficult, but when she began menopause at age 50, her doctor suggested that she not take estrogen plus progestin because of the perceived risks. A bone density test indicated that Beverly had osteopenia, and a blood test identified low vitamin D levels, which is common in women. I recommended she take 600 milligrams of calcium twice daily along with 4,000 milligrams of vitamin D_3 to stave off further bone loss. When Beverly's 25-hydroxy vitamin D levels didn't improve over the following 3 months, I prescribed a 50,000 USP units vitamin D capsule to be taken once a week for 12 weeks. Her vitamin D levels returned to normal, and she kept taking 2,000 units daily to keep her vitamin D levels in the normal range. To gain strength and protect her bones, Beverly also began to walk daily for 30 minutes. Two years later her test showed that her bone density had not gotten worse, which is what we had hoped to achieve.

calcium intake contributes to the development of osteoporosis. Low calcium intake throughout life is associated with low bone mass and high fracture rates.

Eating a diet with calcium-rich foods—dark, oily fish; dark, leafy green vegetables; and low-fat dairy products, for example—is the best way to get the calcium you need. Animal fat not only isn't good for your heart, it isn't good for calcium absorption into bones either. If dietary calcium is not enough, you may need to take a calcium supplement, such as calcium carbonate or calcium citrate. Since most people cannot absorb more than 500 to 600 milligrams at one time, calcium tablets work best when taken throughout the day. Calcium supplements also can cause gas, bloating, and constipation. Calcium citrate has an advantage because you don't have to take it with meals. Calcium carbonate must be taken with meals because eating causes the stomach to produce acid to digest food, and acid is needed to absorb calcium carbonate. Some people chew inexpensive Tums or Rolaids antacid tablets as a source of calcium carbonate.[16] Each pill or chew contains 200 to 400 milligrams of calcium. If you take one of these antacids, add a magnesium and vitamin D supplement and take it with food to increase the acidity of your stomach and improve absorption. Remember, they are antacids, and reduced acid isn't ideal for calcium absorption.

The National Institutes of Health suggest watching out for supplements made from unrefined oyster shell, bonemeal, or dolomite that don't have the USP (United States Pharmacopeia) symbol or the word "purified" on them. They may contain high levels of lead or other toxic metals. Also, be sure to tell your doctor if you take calcium supplements; they can interfere with how your body absorbs certain medications, such as antibiotics and iron pills. Drinking a few glasses of water daily helps your body flush out any "extra" calcium, which lowers the small potential risk of calcium contributing to the formation of kidney stones.

Foods high in oxalic acid, such as spinach, rhubarb, chard, and chocolate, can interfere with calcium absorption by forming insoluble salts in the gut. Foods that contain phytic acid, or phytates, such as whole grains or foods rich in fiber, may reduce the absorption of calcium and other minerals as well. Calcium absorption is improved by protein, fat, and acid foods, but high-protein diets may cause the intestines to increase calcium elimination.[17]

There is, however, a catch when it comes to taking calcium: The body needs vitamin D to absorb calcium. Without enough vitamin D, the body will take calcium stored in the bones, which weakens existing bone and prevents the formation of new bone tissue, resulting in bone loss and osteoporosis. Low amounts of vitamin D also contribute to muscle weakness and may increase the risk of breast, colorectal, prostate, and pancreatic cancers and heart disease.[18, 19] Lack of vitamin D may have an effect on mood, hair, and skin as well and significantly increases the risk of cold and flu.[20] Low levels of vitamin D have been shown to impair sperm production in males and estrogen production in females. Women participants in this study found that they had fewer hot flashes and of less intensity after taking vitamin D supplements that restored their levels to normal. It's important to realize that no matter how important estrogen can be, even during your estrogen window, it's also essential to balance exercise, nutrition, and other lifestyle factors to create a menopause breakthrough.

The body produces a hormone called calcitonin that is secreted by the thyroid gland and reduces the blood calcium level when it rises above normal levels. Calcitonin balances parathyroid hormone, which increases blood calcium levels. Calcitonin lowers calcium by slowing down osteoclasts so they don't break down more bone. A study published in the *Journal of Endocrinological Investigation* indicates that estrogen supplementation in menopausal women increases the levels of calcitonin in the blood.[21] The increase in calcitonin prevented more bone loss in these women than in the group that did not take estrogen. As I've mentioned elsewhere in *The Estrogen Fix*, estrogen works on many parts of the body, not just on the breasts or reproductive organs.

Every week at least one of my patients has low vitamin D levels. Have your 25-hydroxy vitamin D level checked at your next examination with a simple blood test that can change your life. After taking vitamin D_3 supplements, have your blood levels rechecked in 3 months to make sure they are back to normal. (Larger dosages may be required to bring lower levels back to normal.) I suggest that everyone—women and men—take 1,000- to 2,000-IU gelcaps (or other oral supplement) of vitamin D_3 daily, which are available in any pharmacy or health food store (1 microgram of vitamin D_3 equals 40 IU). If you have a low vitamin D level, I recommend that you take vitamin D_3 supplements forever to prevent levels from falling.

While so many people have received the message that using sunscreen can help prevent skin cancer, sunscreens can slow the body's production of vitamin D. Just 20 minutes of sunshine on your hands and face without sunscreen at the beginning or end of the day can help. Then put on your sunscreen.

Estrogen for Osteoporosis

From my point of view, it's always better to prevent a problem than to cure one. That's why my motto is, "It's better to stay well than to get well." For that reason, when estrogen levels begin to drop and your estrogen window opens, it is the perfect time to consider estrogen therapy as a method of osteoporosis prevention. While estrogen is not approved to treat osteoporosis, several estrogen products have been approved to prevent it (see tables to follow). Note that the first table is for women who do not have a uterus and contains ET products only. The second table is for women who do have a uterus and contains EPT products.

Estrogen-Only Medications Approved to Prevent Osteoporosis

MEDICATION	BRAND	HOW SUPPLIED	DOSAGE IN MG
Conjugated estrogens	Premarin	Oral	0.3, 0.45, 0.645, 0.9, 1.25 (daily)
17β-estradiol	Alora	Matrix patch	0.025, 0.05, 0.075, 0.1 (twice/week)
	Climara	Matrix patch	0.025, 0.0375, 0.05, 0.075, 0.1 (once/week)
	Estrace	Oral	0.5, 1.0, 2.0 (daily)
	Menostar	Matrix patch	0.014 (once/week)
	Vivelle	Matrix patch	0.025, 0.0375, 0.05, 0.075, 0.1 (twice/week)
	Vivelle-Dot (Estradot in Canada)	Matrix patch	0.025, 0.0375, 0.05, 0.075, 0.1 (twice/week)
	Estraderm	Reservoir patch	0.05, 0.1 (twice/week)

North American Menopause Society, *Menopause Practice—A Clinician's Guide, 5th Edition*, 2014, p. 130.

EPT Medications Approved to Prevent Osteoporosis

MEDICATION	BRAND	HOW SUPPLIED	DOSAGE IN MG OR μG
Conjugated estrogen (E) + medroxyprogesterone acetate (P) (continuous cyclic)	Premphase	Oral	0.625 mg E + 5.0 mg P/d (E only days 1–14 then E + P days 15–28)
Conjugated estrogen (E) + medroxyprogesterone acetate (P) (continuous combined)	Prempro	Oral	0.3 or 0.45 mg E + 1.5 mg P/d or 0.625 mg E + 2.5 or 5.0 mg P/d (all are 1-tablet combos)
Ethinyl estradiol (E) + norethindrone acetate (P)	Femhrt, femHRT (in Canada)	Oral	2.5 μg E + 1.0 mg P/d or 5.0 μg E + 1.0 mg P/d
17β-estradiol (E) + norethindrone acetate (P)	Activella	Oral	0.5 mg E + 1.0 mg P/d or 1.0 mg E + 0.5 mg P/d
17β-estradiol (E) + norgestimate (P) (intermittent combined)	Prefest	Oral	1.0 mg E + 0.09 mg P (2 tablets E x 3 d then E + P x 3 d, repeatedly)

(continued)

MEDICATION	BRAND	HOW SUPPLIED	DOSAGE IN MG OR μG
17β-estradiol (E) + levonorge-strel (P) (continuous combined)	Climara Pro	Patch	0.045 mg E + 0.015 mg P (22 cm² patch, once/week)
Bazedoxifene (BZA) + conju-gated estrogen (E)	Duavee	Oral	20.0 mg BZA + 0.45 mg E (1 tablet)

North American Menopause Society, *Menopause Practice—A Clinician's Guide*, *5th Edition*, 2014, p. 131.

I've explained why getting a bone density test is essential, but don't wait until bone loss begins to start protecting yourself. Exercise, take vitamin D, eat healthily, and consider taking a low dose of estrogen. It doesn't take very much estrogen to have a huge impact. Even low dosages can prevent bone loss. Despite all the other misgivings, the 2002 WHI study and many others have clearly shown that ET and EPT prevent osteoporosis. If you have a family history of osteoporosis, consider ET or EPT at the beginning of your estrogen window to gain the most benefits and maximize your estrogen fix.

Treatments for Osteoporosis

If you were unable to catch your osteopenia before it turned into osteoporosis, the good news is you still can choose a number of treatments to help stop further bone loss. While taking estrogen is excellent for preventing additional bone loss, it typically won't help build up new bone, especially 3 years after menopause, which is why it's so important to protect your bones when you're young. Most of the other treatments have to do with a relatively new form of treatment called bisphosphonates (see page 151). They can be taken daily, weekly, monthly, or annually. Visit EstrogenFixBook.com for a more complete discussion and a free report on osteoporosis and its treatments that you can download.

One medicine that I want to mention again is Duavee, a new class of medication that combines an estrogen and bazedoxifene (a SERM that protects and builds bone). This may be an excellent way to have some of the benefits of estrogen while specifically blocking most of the worrisome risks. It is approved for the treatment of hot flashes. A recent study found that Duavee improves bone mineral density and at the same time

Lifestyle Changes to Prevent Osteoporosis

- Exercise. If you've been exercising all your life, you've worked hard to maintain your bone health. If you've never exercised, it's not too late to begin. A regular exercise program will help strengthen your bones and muscles and improve your balance and coordination so you can avoid falls and fractures. A regular walking program has been proven to increase bone density in the hips and spine. Choose a combination of weight-bearing and muscle-strengthening exercises. Weight-bearing exercises make you work against gravity while moving in an upright position. Try walking or take a Zumba or exercise class to boost your bone density by 3 to 5 percent per year. Weight-strengthening exercises have you work against gravity while standing, sitting, or lying down. Lifting light weights or using resistance bands (they look like big rubber bands) is ideal.

- Avoid drinking excessive alcohol. Drinking too much alcohol will deplete your body of its calcium reserves and prevent calcium absorption from food. Alcohol hampers liver enzymes that convert inactive vitamin D to the active form. Without sufficient active vitamin D, your body can't absorb calcium from your gastrointestinal tract. Excessive alcohol means more than two drinks of wine, spirits, or beer every day. The

improves vaginal dryness, hot flashes, and quality of life.[22] I think that as time goes by, because of the positive benefits of bazedoxifene, it may be prescribed for a number of other reasons, especially in women who are worried about the risk of breast cancer as Duavee appears to be protective of breast tissue.

A study published in August 2015 in the journal *Menopause* detailed the benefits of bazedoxifene without estrogen in treating midlife women with osteoporosis.[23] After 7 years, the risk of a new fracture of the spine was significantly lower than it was for the placebo group, but the therapy didn't lower the risk of hip fractures, although the hip bone did get significantly denser. The side effects were very minimal and included good news is that some bone loss can be partially restored when excessive drinking is stopped.

- Quit smoking. Studies have shown a connection between smoking and decreased bone density, although researchers aren't sure if decreased bone density is directly related to smoking or to other risk factors in smokers. Smokers tend to be thinner, drink more alcohol, and are less physically active than nonsmokers, putting smokers at increased risk of osteoporosis. Smokers are also at increased risk of breast cancer. The rate of new cases was 24 percent higher in smokers than in nonsmokers and 13 percent higher in former smokers than in nonsmokers.

- Take supplements. Take 1,200 milligrams of calcium, 400 to 800 IU of vitamin D_3 (more vitamin D will be needed if your level is low), and 400 milligrams of magnesium daily. Remember, without vitamin D_3 your body can't absorb calcium.

- Eat a diet rich in calcium and D_3. Eat low-fat dairy products like milk, cottage cheese, and yogurt; dark, leafy greens like kale, arugula, and collard greens; fortified orange juice; and canned sardines and salmon.

some leg cramps and hot flashes. The bazedoxifene did not stimulate the uterine lining or the breast tissue at all. This study helps support the use of Duavee as a combination medication for women who want to consider ET and are worried about breast cancer risk.

Other Medications to Treat Osteoporosis

Bisphosphonates are one of the most common treatments for osteoporosis. They work by inhibiting osteoclasts, the cells that break down bone, so they slow bone loss. These medications must be taken in very specific ways because if they get stuck at the bottom of the esophagus before they enter your stomach, they can cause ulcers in the esophagus. Take them 1 hour or more after getting out of bed in the morning, drink lots of water, and remain in an upright position for 30 to 60 minutes.

Actonel, Binosto, Boniva, and Fosamax. These are available as brand names or as generic medications. Actonel, Binosto, and Fosamax are usually taken once a week; Boniva is taken once a month.

Reclast is another bisphosphonate that is given via a 15-minute infusion in a vein once each year. The benefit of Reclast is that it increases bone strength and reduces fractures in the hip, spine, wrist, arm, leg, and rib.

SERMs

Evista is a selective estrogen receptor modulator or SERM, which is similar to an estrogen but acts differently in different tissues. The goal is for the SERM to stimulate the bone or take other positive actions and spare or block the estrogen impact on the breast and uterine lining where potential harm could take place. Evista treats osteoporosis similar to the way estrogen does in its ability to maintain bone mass, but it doesn't increase the risk of breast or uterine cancers. Evista can cause blood clots and often causes some hot flashes.

Parathyroid Hormone

Forteo is a synthetic parathyroid, and its real name is teriparatide. It is used to treat osteoporosis in postmenopausal women and men who are at high risk of a fracture. Forteo is the first drug shown to stimulate new bone formation and increase bone mineral density. It has to be taken daily as an injection you give to yourself for up to 24 months and can cause nausea, leg cramps, and dizziness.

Synthetic Molecules

Prolia (denosumab) is a very specific synthetic type of substance called a monoclonal antibody that blocks the effect of osteoclasts.[24] It is a type of "biological treatment" approved to treat postmenopausal women with osteoporosis and high risk of fracture, and when other osteoporosis medicines have not worked.

Chapter 8

The Estrogen Fix and Your Vagina, Bladder, and Skin

You may find the grouping of vagina, bladder, and skin somewhat unusual. But as you read on, you will see that they do share quite a bit in common as far as their relationship to estrogen and the estrogen window and your estrogen fix. As explained in previous chapters, taking estrogen during your estrogen window offers major benefits to the brain, heart, bones, and breasts. You may be surprised to learn that estrogen can also have a positive effect on maintaining vaginal and bladder health as well as keeping your skin looking more youthful.

As one woman told me, "When I was young, my skin was smooth and my vagina was wrinkled; now my face is wrinkled and my vagina is smooth." These changes are largely due to changes in estrogen levels. Lower estrogen levels can make sexual intercourse uncomfortable, contribute to urinary tract infections and incontinence, and cause loss of the collagen that keeps facial skin smooth, plump, and youthful. Although the estrogen window has a very specific opening and closing for the brain, heart, breasts, and bones, estrogen can continue to impart some benefits to the skin and bladder after the estrogen window closes; the estrogen window for the vagina stays open, though in severe cases of vaginal narrowing, it may not be able to return completely back to the premenopausal state.

The Estrogen Fix and Vaginal Tissue

Vaginal tissue has unique characteristics. It allows menstrual flow to pass through it without absorbing it. It creates pleasure through sexual intercourse, is tight enough to bring pleasure to your partner, and expands widely enough to permit a baby to pass through it.

During a woman's reproductive years, the walls of the vagina are corrugated, like the elastic ribbing of a sock, which allows the tissue to expand and return to its original size. When you are lying down, your bladder sits on top of the vagina and your rectum lies below it. Your cervix, the "neck" of your uterus, lies at the top of it. The vagina is filled with bacteria, including lactobacillus and other "good" bacteria, and some E. coli and other "bad" bacteria that are balanced when the vaginal pH, or level of acidity, is kept relatively constant at 3.5 to 4.5. Estrogen maintains this acidic pH. Here's how: Before menopause, estrogen causes the outer layer of vaginal cells to shed naturally. When these cells die, they cause the release of glycogen that in turn is converted to glucose or sugar. The "good" lactobacillus bacteria convert the glucose to lactic acid, which is acid and keeps the healthy premenopausal pH between 3.5 and 4.5.[1] It's the same ecological concept as when leaves fall from trees in the autumn and change the pH of the soil around them. As estrogen levels decline in perimenopause and menopause, this process becomes less active, and vaginal pH begins to rise to levels that range from 5.0 to 7.5. At these pH levels, the lactobacillus can't survive as well, and so-called bad bacteria begin to change the balance, a condition called *atrophic vaginitis*. That sets the stage for menopausal women to have more symptomatic vaginal and urinary tract infections.[2, 3]

With aging, the loss of estrogen, and changes in vaginal pH and bacteria, the vaginal walls thin and weaken along with some of the surrounding muscles and ligaments, which allows the bladder to drop down and the rectum to push forward. The corrugated "wrinkles" of the vagina, called rugae (ROO-guy), begin to flatten, and the walls begin to smooth out. The end result is that the once "elastic" vagina becomes more rigid. Lack of estrogen also causes the vaginal bloodflow to lessen, which changes the color of the vagina from pink to pale and reduces moisture. Over time, the tissue narrows and shortens, and that can lead to painful intercourse,[4] vaginal dryness, occasional bleeding, and just plain discomfort. If you've ever noticed slight bleeding after a pelvic examination or intercourse, this could be the reason. The good news is that it doesn't happen to every woman, though it is extremely common.[5] The bad news is that only about 25 percent of women who have symptoms of vaginal atrophy ask their health-care provider for help.[6] In fact, it remains undertreated among all postmenopausal age groups.[7]

This does not have to be part of "normal aging," and you shouldn't have to endure it. Unlike hot flashes that eventually go away, these symptoms usually get worse over time and increase from early menopause to late menopause.[8] While it's possible that your doctor may think you have a vaginal infection caused by yeast or bacteria, know that is only one possibility. It could also be part of an ongoing process that can be stopped and easily reversed with estrogen once you start treatment. In contrast to estrogen for breasts, bones, brain, and heart, the ability of the vagina to respond almost completely once the estrogen window closes means that the vagina's estrogen window stays open for an estrogen fix.

Because the term *vaginal atrophy* sounds so negative (more than one of my patients has said, "It makes me sound like I'm all shriveled up"), the North American Menopause Society and the Society for Sexual Medicine have suggested that the condition be renamed *genitourinary syndrome of menopause* (GSM). The term *vaginal atrophy* is just starting to be replaced by the newer term. I'm glad my colleagues realize that sensitivity is needed, and what we call this condition has an impact on how women feel when they talk about it with their doctors.

After the Women's Health Initiative (WHI) report was published in 2002 showing possible risks from estrogen, women in and around menopause stopped using estrogen to treat their hot flashes, osteoporosis, and heart disease. Without the benefits of estrogen on the vaginal tissues, one-third of women began to experience genitourinary syndrome of menopause, which included symptoms of vaginal dryness, irritation, itching, and/or painful sex (dyspareunia).[9] Although some women find that continued sexual activity with a partner or alone can help keep the tissues healthy because of increased bloodflow, the low estrogen and resulting vaginal dryness can require much more time to lubricate before intercourse, and even then the vagina may not produce enough moisture to avoid discomfort, even if you're ready and full of desire. It can be very challenging to be "in the mood" if you know sex is going to hurt. The unfortunate thing is that because the symptoms typically first show up

SANDRA is 54 years old and in a loving relationship with her husband. Before menopause they had an active sex life and had relations two or three times per week. For 3 years Sandra noticed she had less interest in sex than she used to, but with more foreplay, she found herself able to get into the mood and achieve an orgasm. Over the last 2 years, sexual intercourse became excruciatingly painful. No matter how long they spent on foreplay, as soon as her husband entered her she felt like her vagina was on fire, and when he ejaculated, the seminal fluid caused her vagina to burn just as badly. "It hurt so bad," she told me, "I'd rather be shopping. And he feels terrible because he thinks it's his fault and is hurting me. Sometimes I just tell him it's okay and go ahead. But having an orgasm isn't going to happen for me. I just want to satisfy him. I'm afraid if he doesn't get what he wants at home, he'll go find it somewhere else—and at this point, I wouldn't blame him."

Taking the time to explain to Sandra what was happening to her body and prescribing her vaginal estrogen allowed her to return to a satisfactory, and eventually a satisfying, relationship with her husband in just a few weeks.

I've heard this complaint from women so many times. I also explained to Sandra that once she started taking estrogen, sexual intercourse might be initially uncomfortable, as she hadn't been sexually active for some time. Like any muscle, the vaginal tissues have to "get back in shape," which could take a week or two after HT is started.

several years after menopause, many women don't realize that their symptoms are due to menopause and don't realize it is a medical problem that can be easily treated. I want you to know that you don't have to grin and bear vaginal dryness and discomfort.

Low estrogen levels at midlife also reduce bloodflow to the clitoris, the introitus (the entry to the vagina), and the labia (the "lips" or folds around the opening of the vagina). Those changes can cause pain when a penis or sex toy enters the vagina and reduce sensation as the outer tissues begin to shrink. This is explained in greater detail when I explain how low estrogen affects the urinary tract tissues.

Estrogen taken either orally, transdermally, or inserted into the vagina can often improve these symptoms.[10, 11] This use of vaginal estrogen is so beneficial that when vaginal surgery, such as repair of a cystocele (when the bladder drops into the vagina because of weakening of the tissues around the vagina), is performed on women in menopause, local estrogen is often prescribed beforehand to build up the vaginal tissues. The process is more successful because the tissue is stronger and healthier before the surgery, so the healing and results are improved.

In the discussion of the estrogen window and your skin (page 165), the tissue of the skin and the lining of the vagina have more in common than you might think. I have performed surgery on a number of young women who were born without vaginas, a condition known as Mayer-Rokitansky-Küster-Hauser syndrome. These women typically have their uterus and ovaries, so the procedure is done around the time of puberty to create a channel for menstrual tissue to leave their bodies. The surgery, called a McIndoe procedure, is done by making an incision where the vagina is supposed to be. Skin is then shaved from a buttock or thigh to be used as a graft. That skin graft is placed around a piece of balsa wood shaped to size to use as a mold to shape the future vagina. The mold with the skin around it is then sewn into the incision where the vagina would form. A week or two later the mold is removed and the young woman is taught how to keep her new vagina open with a dilator. After several months, the skin graft looks exactly like normal vaginal tissue. Amazingly, once in the right location, the skin when exposed to estrogen produced by the body becomes normal vaginal tissue.

Using Estrogen Vaginally

Since 1918 it has been common knowledge that medications ranging from morphine to estrogen can be absorbed through the vaginal walls.[12] While much of the medicine remains local, depending on what the medication is and the dosage, drugs placed into the vagina can reach therapeutic blood levels throughout the body.

Taking medication vaginally rather than orally means side effects such as vomiting, variable absorption from the intestines, and certain drug interactions can be avoided. Taking a medicine through the skin, or transdermally, avoids some of these potential problems, but you still have to take into account how much fat a person has on her body, because the amount of fat changes the amount of absorption—the more you weigh, the less of the medication you may absorb. As mentioned in other chapters, taking estrogen or other medications vaginally means they avoid passing through the liver, which can have an impact on the amount of medication absorbed, distributed, and excreted.[13] A vaginal delivery system can result in a steadier release of medication into your bloodstream and have fewer side effects. It can also provide a way to get hormones to the uterus and pelvic organs through local bloodflow.[14]

Sometimes taking estrogen orally or transdermally will provide adequate levels to your body but supply lesser concentrations to the vaginal tissues. Women who take oral and transdermal estrogen may also require a local estrogen to help the vagina. In contrast, taking estrogen locally in lower concentrations can provide an adequate amount of estrogen to the vagina and to a slightly lesser extent to the pelvic organs, but *much* lower concentrations to the bloodstream and rest of the body. So realize that oral or transdermal estrogen, particularly low dosages, may need supplementation to be optimally effective for the vaginal tissues. Most of the estrogen placed into the vagina remains in the pelvic tissues, but some, depending on which type and what dosage you use, will likely get into the bloodstream.

Some women express concern that medication taken vaginally will leak out. In reality, when a woman is standing, the vagina is in a mostly horizontal position. I've never had a patient complain that a vaginal tablet or suppository fell out. Small amounts of a cream may escape onto the lips of the vagina (vulva), which is a good thing for treating the tissues just outside the vagina. Many women worry that taking vaginal estrogen isn't safe, especially if they read the black box warning currently required by the FDA stating that estrogen can cause breast cancer, heart attacks, dementia, and more. The reality is that there is no evidence that vaginal estrogen in dosages designed to relieve vaginal dryness cause any risk for these medical conditions. There is some absorption into the bloodstream, but as I mentioned in Chapter 3, it is an extremely small amount. In fact, the American College of Obstetricians and Gynecologists published a Committee Opinion in March 2016 stating that "while non-hormonal approaches should be tried first . . . women with a history of estrogen-dependent breast cancer who are experiencing urogenital symptoms can use vaginal estrogen . . . because the data do not show an increased risk of cancer recurrence among women currently undergoing treatment for breast cancer or those with a personal history of breast cancer."[15] In other words, there is no need to suffer if you have vaginal pain.

To continue receiving the benefits of vaginal estrogen, you have to keep taking it on an ongoing basis. If you do stop treatment, within a few months, the vaginal and surrounding tissues will return to the state they were in before you started the medication. If you stop taking local estrogen, you can always start again; although as time passes, the vagina becomes narrower and shorter and the response to local estrogen may be a little less effective. As previously mentioned, unlike the estrogen window for brain, breasts, bones, and heart, the estrogen window for vaginal tissues always remains open and the estrogen fix is always possible.

One often overlooked point is that low estrogen levels that lead to genitourinary syndrome of menopause can make it challenging for a health-care practitioner to do a comfortable and thorough annual pelvic examination, especially on women who are well into their seventies, eighties, or beyond. As a result, diagnosing the cause of certain symptoms, such as vaginal bleeding, can be challenging. This is another reason to consider inserting small amounts of estrogen into the vagina even if you are not sexually active and have genitourinary syndrome of menopause. It's another benefit of the estrogen fix.

There are several ways to use vaginal estrogen, depending on your preferences: pills, creams, or rings. Here is a summary of those options.

VAGINAL TYPE	TYPE OF ESTROGEN (BRAND)	DOSING
Creams	Conjugated equine estrogen (CEE) (Premarin—0.625 mg/g active ingredient) and estradiol (Estrace—0.1 mg/g active ingredient)	Typically taken 0.5–2.0 grams daily for 21 days followed by 7 days off; or 0.5–2 grams twice per week; estradiol typically given 2–4 grams daily for 1–2 weeks then 1 gram 1–3 times weekly for maintenance
Ring (Estring)[16]	2-mg estradiol reservoir designed for vaginal symptoms	Releases ~7.5 µg daily for 90 days, then removed and replaced
Tablet (Vagifem)[17]	10 µg estradiol equivalent—ultra-low-dose of estradiol hemihydrate	1 tablet daily for 2 weeks, then one tablet twice weekly
Femring[18]	Delivers total body levels of estradiol, far more than Estring, comparable to pills and patches	Contains either 12.4 mg or 24.8 mg. Usually lasts for 3 months, then removed and replaced, releases either 0.05 mg/day or 0.1 mg/day

North American Menopause Society, *Menopause Practice—A Clinician's Guide.*
5th Edition, 2014, p. 267.

In November 2016, the US Food and Drug Administration approved Intrarosa (prasterone) to treat women who have moderate to severe pain during sexual intercourse (dyspareunia), due to vulvar and vaginal atrophy (VVA) or genitourinary syndrome of menopause (GSM). Intrarosa is the first FDA approved product containing the active ingredient prasterone, which is also known as dehydroepiandrosterone (DHEA). It's given as a once a day vaginal insert.

There is also a new vaginal estradiol gel cap called VagiCap that is currently being investigated under the name of TX-004HR. It is used once daily for 2 weeks and then twice per week. Dosages of 25 micrograms, 10 micrograms, and 4 micrograms were studied, and all resulted is statistically significant improvement in vaginal tissue and in symptoms. This medication will likely become FDA approved with the year.

The Estrogen Fix and Your Bladder

If you know where every bathroom is located along your everyday routes, in every mall, and in all the office buildings you frequent, you already know that having a sensitive bladder can be one of the most challenging symptoms of menopause. And it can be downright embarrassing. A sensitive bladder can be even worse if urine leaks every time you cough, laugh, exercise, sneeze, or make love. And urinary tract infections (UTIs) can be a real pain, both literally and figuratively. Estrogen plays an important role in the female urinary tract and tissues, particularly the bladder and the urethra (the tube from the bladder that urine passes out through), just as it does in the brain, breasts, bones, and other organs.[19]

About half of women have urine leakage at some point in their lives, and for many it's a daily problem.[20] And while it is more common around menopause and beyond, that doesn't mean you have to put up with it. Unless you have a UTI, urine loss is not a disease—it's a problem. The problem is so embarrassing that women feel shame or may even think incontinence is a normal and inevitable part of aging, so they often wait between 5 and 7 years before telling their health-care providers that they have a problem.[21]

I mentioned earlier that thinning of the vaginal tissues and surrounding muscles and ligaments due to decreased estrogen may cause the bladder to "drop," and that can be one reason for frequent urination, a "leaky" bladder, or other urinary tract issues in menopause. That is particularly true if the pelvic tissues have been damaged from childbirth. But estrogen plays a more direct role on the bladder as well.[22]

Think of the bladder as a balloon. Urine filters through the kidneys into tubes called ureters that in turn enter two sides of the bladder into a triangle-shaped muscle called the trigone. At the bottom of the trigone is another opening that leads to the urethra, where the urine exits. The trigone keeps urine in the bladder until it reaches a certain pressure, and then nerves in the area tell your brain it's time to urinate. You control your trigone until you get to the bathroom, and then the trigone relaxes and lets urine flow out.

Lower estrogen levels can weaken the bladder's trigone muscle, weaken the surrounding tissues, and affect the closing pressure of the urethra and how well a woman can tell if her bladder is getting full.[23] And all this contributes to less bladder control and a more sensitive bladder.[24] This is another explanation for why estrogen and the estrogen window play important, in this case supporting, roles when it comes to bladder issues, and why you may benefit from an estrogen fix. Menopause also contributes to urinary tract problems because the lining of the urethra, the fascia (surrounding canvas), and the pelvic muscles may weaken when estrogen levels decline, causing involuntary loss of urine. Taking estrogen can reverse some of these changes, though depending on how much tissue loss has occurred, it may not be possible to return everything back to the premenopausal state. (To determine how your bladder symptoms compare with those of other women and some tips on what to do about them, visit MenopauseQuiz.com.)

Involuntary loss of urine (incontinence) is a major problem for American men and women. To get an idea of how many adults struggle with bladder control, walk into any drugstore. Shelves are stacked with packages of adult absorption pads, such as Depend, and more are sold each year than disposable baby diapers.

Half of all menopausal women will experience some urinary incontinence, and 25 percent will require surgery to correct it. It is one of the most embarrassing aspects of aging. It's easy to understand why most women wait 5 to 7 years to tell their doctors that they are having a problem. The good news is that 75 percent of urinary tract problems can be improved or corrected through nonsurgical approaches such as medications and biofeedback.

Women are more likely to suffer from urinary incontinence than men.

The urethra—the tube that carries urine from the bladder out of the body—is shorter in women than it is in men. In addition, pregnancy and childbirth can weaken the pelvic muscles and fascia, the canvas sheath that reinforces and additionally supports the urethra. Women who have had children are more likely to experience involuntary urine loss than those who have not.

The North American Menopause Society's *Menopause Guidebook* notes that UTIs of the bladder (cystitis); other medical conditions such as multiple sclerosis; certain prescription drugs, such as diuretics and some tranquilizers; smoking; eating spicy foods and artificial sweeteners; or drinking alcohol and caffeine can irritate the bladder and make incontinence worse. Acidic foods like tomatoes and fruit juices can contribute to the problem.

Studies have demonstrated that estrogen has been helpful to 40 to 70 percent of women with urinary incontinence.[25] I recommend that my patients use vaginal estrogen cream, which I believe works better than tablets or patches for urinary incontinence. One-fourth to one-half of a full applicator of estrogen cream is inserted into the vagina daily for 2 weeks and then once or twice a week after that. After 3 months, the tissue usually regains much of its strength, and the medication can be reduced or used less often. Performing Kegel exercises while using the vaginal cream also helps. If you do try this approach, your breasts and nipples may feel full or even tingle because some of the estrogen will be

MY mother, who is 93, phoned to tell me she was feeling very tired, had a little backache, and thought her "arthritis was acting up." She said urination was just a little uncomfortable, she hadn't been drinking much water, and she didn't have a fever. It was a Friday afternoon. I asked her to start drinking several glasses of water and go in to see her doctor right then to check for a UTI. She did have a UTI. In addition to taking an antibiotic, she was told to drink six to eight glasses of water. The next day she felt so much better. In 2 days she felt like herself. So often people, especially the elderly, don't drink enough water, which contributes to UTIs and dehydration. I told her to put a pitcher of water on her drain board and drink it between breakfast and dinner so she know she consumed 2 quarts of water a day. She also started using a small amount of vaginal estrogen, which has made her feel much more comfortable.

absorbed into your bloodstream. I cover sensitive bladder in more detail in my webinar at MenopauseBreakthrough.com.

Urinary Tract Infections (UTIs)

First you experienced vaginal dryness and uncomfortable sex, and now you find yourself suffering repeatedly from UTIs, which can be painful. Once again you can look to lower estrogen levels during perimenopause and menopause for contributing to these problems.

As we've discussed, women's vaginal tissues and urinary tracts are sensitive to estrogen. As a woman transitions from her reproductive years into perimenopause and menopause, less estrogen is available to those tissues, which causes the symptoms of perimenopause and menopause. When estrogen is abundant during the reproductive years, the end of the urethra—the tiny tube that carries urine out of the bladder—typically is level with the tissues of the upper vagina and is protected from infection. As menopause approaches and estrogen levels become lower, the vagina shortens and narrows, and outer vaginal tissues pull back from the tip of the urethra. That leaves the tip of the urethra exposed to more bacteria and at a higher risk of infection. UTI symptoms include burning when urinating, going to the bathroom frequently, cloudy urine, occasionally back or flank pain, and sometimes a fever.

If you are going through perimenopause or menopause and are experiencing frequent UTIs, talk with your health-care provider about what approach is best for you. If left untreated, a UTI can lead to serious consequences. Some of my elderly patients develop UTIs that become a silent cause of sepsis, or a total body infection.

More than half of women will have a UTI in their lifetime, and about 25 to 30 percent of those women will be younger than 55 years old. For women 55 or older, the chance of developing a recurring UTI increases. More than half of those women who experience a UTI will get another UTI within 6 to 12 months.

Despite a greater risk of developing a UTI during menopause because of lower estrogen levels, there are things you can do about it. Here are the best ways to lower your risk of getting a UTI during perimenopause and menopause:

1. **Take low-dose estrogen**. Low-dose estrogen in the form of a tablet, cream, suppository, or vaginal ring is a very effective way to help

prevent recurring UTIs. When estrogen is applied locally (directly to the reproductive or outer vaginal tissues), it *mostly* stays in the vaginal area. Most forms do seep into the bloodstream somewhat, but the amount is small and the risks minimal, even if you have breast cancer (as I mentioned above). So discuss this with your health-care provider. Vaginal estrogen also seeps into the bladder, which can strengthen the cells of the bladder lining. One study[26] found that for women with recurring UTIs, both local estrogen and antibiotics reduced UTIs per year by roughly half. In another study of postmenopausal women with more than three UTIs in the prior year, treating them with Estring for 36 weeks resulted in 45 percent not having a recurrent infection compared with 20 percent taking a placebo.[27] And both oral and vaginal estrogen have been shown to significantly increase blood-flow to the vagina, bladder, and urethra.[28] The estrogen works in two ways: (1) by building up the tissues within and just outside the vagina, which protects the urethra from exposure to more bacteria, and (2) by stimulating production of the body's own antibiotic in the lining cells of the bladder. Early action by the bladder's internal defense mechanism reduces the number of bacteria before they have a chance to multiply enough to cause an infection. Estrogen therapy also improves women's vaginal dryness and painful sex[29] without contributing to antibiotic resistance, which is why local estrogen is my first choice for preventing recurrent UTIs during menopause. If you want to know whether your estrogen levels are high enough to prevent painful intercourse, here is some practical information: Women whose estradiol levels are > 50 pg/mL have less vaginal dryness and painful sex during intercourse. Women whose estradiol levels are < 35 pg/mL report less sexual activity.[30, 31]

One final point: In a substudy of the WHI, treatment with conjugated estrogen plus progestin resulted in an increase in stress incontinence, which is loss of urine with coughing or sneezing. But in women 59 or younger, there was no significant increase of stress incontinence.[32] And in a review article of 35 other articles on stress incontinence, there was a 64 to 75 percent improvement in stress incontinence with oral and/or vaginal estrogen therapy.[33] So just as is true for breasts, brain, bones, and heart, there is an estrogen window for stress incontinence and the estrogen fix.

2. **Control or correct other medical conditions.** Women with type 2 diabetes or sensitive bladder issues, such as difficulty emptying their bladder, are at an increased risk of UTIs. Controlling blood sugar if you have diabetes, or correcting bladder problems, can help lower the risk of UTIs.

3. **Eat foods rich in probiotics.** Instead of trying to kill "bad bacteria," some studies suggest putting "good bacteria" into the pelvic organs to re-create balance. Taking medications with lactobacillus, a type of good bacteria, twice daily is helpful. The higher the concentration of lactobacillus, the better it is for you. Compare labels and get the option with the most lactobacillus or "good" bacteria in it. Fermented foods, such as sauerkraut, kimchi (pickled cabbage), kefir, sour pickles, and miso soup, and supplements such as Culturelle and RepHresh Pro-B are good sources of probiotics. Yogurts that contain the National Yogurt Association's "Live and Active Cultures" (LAC) seal contain at least 100 million LACs per gram at the time of manufacture. Look for the words "active culture," "live culture," or "live active culture" on the label.

4. **Make small changes to your daily life.** Lower your risk of developing a UTI during perimenopause or menopause by staying hydrated and drinking plenty of water; wiping front to back when you use the bathroom; avoiding irritating feminine products like douches, powders, and deodorant sprays; and wearing cotton underwear to keep the area dry.

5. **Urinate regularly.** "Holding it" is never good. Not only is it uncomfortable, but it can also make it easier for bacteria to multiply in your urinary tract. Urinating before and after sexual intercourse can also prevent bacteria from moving into the urethra.

6. **Take antibiotics as a last resort.** Try using these previous methods as much as possible, because frequent antibiotic use can cause bacterial resistance. For that reason, using long-term antibiotics to prevent UTIs is becoming less popular today.

Estrogen and Your Skin

When women are asked what is most bothersome about menopause, answers such as hot flashes, vaginal dryness, weight gain, or lower

How to Take Care of Your Skin

Since skin damage can be caused by too much exposure to the sun, smoking, and other environmental substances as well as estrogen loss, cosmetic dermatologist Dr. Dina Anderson suggests some non-estrogen approaches to skin care:

- Use sunscreen every day. It is never too late to start using sunscreen, especially on your face. SPF 15 filters out 93 percent of UVB, and SPF 30 filters out 97 percent. There is no rating to tell you how good a sunscreen is at blocking UVA. The best ingredients to block UVA are ecamsule, avobenzone, oxybenzone, titanium dioxide, or zinc oxide, so look for them on the packaging.

- Try a topical retinoid. Topical retinoids, such as Retin-A, shut off proteins called matrix metalloproteinases that break down collagen. According to Dr. Anderson, retinoids also normalize cells called melanocytes, which reduce blotchiness and help bring more bloodflow to the skin to counter the loss of estrogen. Retinols require a prescription, and the directions should be followed carefully.

- Try other topical skin care. Substances such as topical resveratrol, topical green tea, topical caffeine, and topical stable vitamin C all work well to protect against free radicals and decrease oxidative stress, which will make your skin healthier.

- Eat food rich in omega-3s. Anything that decreases inflammation and oxidative stress, such as avoiding processed foods

sex drive are common. But the universal concerns on the minds of most women when the word *menopause* is mentioned is getting and looking older. And since the skin is the body's largest organ—the one literally staring us in the face—skin, facial in particular, has special meaning to women.

According to the American Society for Aesthetic Plastic Surgery's March 11, 2015, press release, Americans spent more than 12 billion dollars on surgical and nonsurgical procedures for the second year in a and trans fats and eating foods rich in omega-3s (wild, oily fish such as halibut, salmon, and sardines; grains; nuts; and dark, leafy greens), will help your skin look healthier.

• Lower your stress levels and get plenty of uninterrupted sleep. These do contribute to healthy skin by lowering the "stress" hormone cortisol. It's all part of creating a complete lifestyle approach that allows you to live a healthy life to its fullest.

• Consider cosmetic treatments. A number of cosmetic dermatological treatments result in younger-looking skin, depending on how much time and money you're willing to spend. Glycolic peels at a dermatologist's office can improve the skin's surface, texture, and tone. Fraxel laser treatments smooth out some fine lines, get rid of brown spots, and make the skin look more youthful. Injectable therapies, including fillers and Botox, can help restructure the skin and support tissues that depleted during menopause. We've all seen the faces of celebrities and others who have gone too far with facial treatments and cosmetic surgeries. If you want to look 5 to 10 years younger than you do now, that's entirely possible, but don't expect to regain your youth with injections and cosmetic procedures. Utilizing your estrogen window will reduce and delay the need for these types of treatments and provides an estrogen fix.

row. Most of the procedures were done on women, who enhanced, increased, or decreased their eyelids, faces, chins, tummies, breasts, buttocks, noses, and even their vaginal and vulva tissues.[34] Looks matter, and estrogen plays an important role.

It is known that applying estrogen topically to the skin can improve age-related changes such as wrinkles and thin skin. That is largely because the skin is rich in alpha and beta estrogen receptors that make it highly responsive to estrogen. I mentioned earlier in this chapter that

DURING her annual examination, 63-year-old Delfina shared this with me: "I keep a file of packing lists for my travels, so I make sure to bring all the medications and other products. I found a list from when I was in my early forties reminding me to pack Loestrin, a low-dose birth control pill, which I took every day, and estradiol, which I took for the first 10 days of the month. Since I was a pack-a-day cigarette smoker until I was in my late thirties, I went into early menopause around 40. I clearly remember that while taking Loestrin and estradiol, people frequently commented on my beautiful, plump, youthful facial skin. When I stopped taking the pills 12 years later, my skin began to look and feel awful—pitted as if I had acne, no elasticity, and dry. How I wish I could take estrogen again just for those benefits!"

surgeons use estrogen to strengthen vaginal tissues before certain operations. Estrogen has also been used to improve the healing of skin wounds in older women and men. Estrogen acts by lowering inflammation, bringing in new blood vessels, and generally helping wounds heal.[35] This is similar to what happens in the brain, heart, and bones. Using estrogen seems to be somewhat less effective after age 70 because the estrogen receptors in the skin become significantly reduced at that time.[36]

All this has an impact on how "good" you look, how old you look, and the quality of your skin as you age. Just like vaginal tissues become less elastic with aging, the tissues of the face and skin are also going through "the change."[37] Around and beyond menopause, lower levels of estrogen are associated with the fine wrinkles that appear on skin, thinning of the outer layer of the skin, and progressive loss of the collagen layer under the skin that serves as a scaffolding to keep the skin stretched and smooth. The skin also becomes less moist, begins to sag, and doesn't heal as quickly or as well as it once did. Estrogen restores skin thickness by increasing collagen synthesis while at the same time limiting collagen loss. Estrogen also helps reduce wrinkles by increasing elastic fibers under the skin and another component of the skin's scaffolding—hyaluronic acid. Estrogen helps the skin retain water, which increases moisture, encourages natural oil production, and lowers inflammation.

When you compare the skin of postmenopausal women taking estrogen with those who are not, there are some significant differences. Within 6 months of taking oral estrogen, the skin is thicker.[38] Topical estrogen can achieve these results in as little as 2 weeks.[39] When postmenopausal women who have taken estrogen since menopause for 5 years are compared with women who have not taken estrogen for the first 5 years after menopause, the women who take estrogen have significantly fewer wrinkles.[40] Simply stated, estrogen improves the detrimental skin changes of aging on the face and body.

Women not taking estrogen lose 1.13 percent of skin thickness and 2 percent of their collagen every year after menopause.[41] Type I and type III skin collagen is believed to reduce by up to 30 percent in the first 5 years after menopause,[42] which is comparable to the rate of bone loss that occurs after menopause.[43] As with the estrogen window in other parts of the body, the decrease in skin thickness and collagen content correlates more with years since menopause than the age of the woman.[44, 45] All this has a great impact on appearance. Randomized, double-blind, placebo-controlled studies have shown that 1 year of oral estrogen can increase skin thickness by 30 percent[46] if taken early, and increase collagen 6.49 percent in 6 months.[47] The more collagen a woman has at the time she begins taking estrogen, the more effective the estrogen will be in maintaining or increasing her collagen levels; so the closer to menopause estrogen is begun, the greater the impact will be.[48]

Although applying estrogen cream topically has been investigated for decades,[49] I'm not promoting the idea of slathering estrogen all over your face. It is an interesting notion, and both topical estradiol (Estrace) and conjugated estrogen (Premarin) cream have been studied. Topical estrogen only seems to be effective in the areas to which it is applied. In addition, topical estrogen applied to your face is transdermal estrogen and will travel to all parts of your body, so dosing has to be monitored so as not to raise blood levels more than desired. However, because I've taken care of so many women who come to me with what I call "myth-information" about the overall safety of estrogen if taken during the estrogen window, I know that they have experienced many of the symptoms of menopause, including early aging of their face and skin. Given the amount of plastic surgery taking place these days, this information is important to many women. I am aware of research being done on an estrogen that is intended to be applied to the skin to treat wrinkles, and this estrogen actually breaks down into inactive substances before entering the bloodstream. This could be an exciting new way for women to address their skin concerns without increasing blood levels of estrogen for those who don't want to take or apply it.

At an annual meeting of the North American Menopause Society, I interviewed New York cosmetic dermatologist Dr. Dina Anderson for *The Hot Years-My Menopause Magazine* about how aging and lower estrogen levels associated with menopause impact a woman's appearance. She revealed that these changes can begin when a woman is in her thirties, depending on how young she is when she begins to transition into menopause. A young woman's face typically looks like an inverted triangle—it's wide across the forehead, begins to narrow at the cheeks, and is "pointed" at the chin.

Lower estrogen levels lead to a loss of collagen and other substances that at younger ages keep a face looking smooth and youthful. With estrogen's decline, fine lines become visible and the fat pads of the temples, forehead, and cheeks begin to separate and reduce in size, causing the face to appear a bit hollow. Like other bones in the body, first the bones in the face begin to thin and the orbits of the eyes and cheekbones contract. Then the bone that supports the jawline shrinks. When that happens, in addition to fine lines, wrinkles, and crow's-feet around the eyes, the face begins to sag. The overall shape of the face that once looked like an inverted triangle now begins to look like a triangle with the point at the top and base at the bottom. Just like breasts and midriffs sag, so does the face.

As a result, women in their midfifties often say, "My eyelids kind of fall over my eyes." And the two skin folds that run from each side of the nose to the corners of your mouth, the so-called "smile lines" or "laugh lines," start to hang over because the bone is contracted.

Now you understand why estrogen has such powerful and positive effects on so many aspects of a woman's health and wellness when her estrogen window is open and an estrogen fix is most likely—and while the skin and the bladder do have a specific estrogen window, for the vagina the estrogen window remains open unless genitourinary syndrome of menopause is extreme.

Chapter 9

The Estrogen Fix for a Fit, Energized Body

Love handles. Muffin top. Spare tire. Menopot. Jelly belly. The list of disparaging terms women use for the belly fat from menopause goes on and on. As they stare into the mirror at their once-svelte bodies and try to zip up a favorite pair of pants, they wonder what is going on. "I've got a closet full of clothes that don't fit," one of my patients told me, "and I don't get it! I go to the gym four times a week and eat a pretty healthy diet. I cut way back on carbs like pasta and bread and treat myself to a glass of wine just twice a week, but nothing I do makes any difference. If I lose weight, it's from my face, neck, and arms, but not from my waist and belly."

Belly fat is not just a cosmetic issue, limited to the amount of fat we can pinch between our fingers; it also has a more sinister medical significance. Another accumulation of fat surrounds our internal organs beneath the fascia or canvas covering of our belly: visceral fat. It really should be called "vicious" fat because it contributes to a host of diseases that increase the risk of heart disease, high blood pressure, stroke, joint disease, and type 2 diabetes,[1] though for 16 percent of women, their metabolism stays healthy in spite of their increased weight,[2] probably because of genetic factors.[3] Studies show that being overweight or obese isn't only a medical issue; it also affects quality of life and self-esteem.[4]

Body Mass Index (BMI)

Body mass index (BMI) is a person's weight in kilograms divided by the square of height in meters. A high BMI can be an indicator of high body fat. BMI is a screening tool, but it does not diagnose fatness or health of an individual.

To calculate your BMI, use the BMI calculator at: http://1.usa .gov/1dSzT3p.

- A BMI less than 18.5 falls within the underweight range.

- A BMI 18.5 to 24.9 falls within the normal or healthy weight range.

- A BMI 25.0 to 29.9 falls within the overweight range.

- A BMI 30.0 or higher falls within the obese range.

I have a personal appreciation for this issue. When I was helping my then 91-year-old mother move from the house I grew up in to a smaller condominium, I found a box of old newspapers. In that box were the headlines "Pearl Harbor Attacked" and "President Kennedy Assassinated." But it was a different front-page headline that caught my attention; it read, "Mighty Might: The Fattest Kid in the County." The photo was taken many years ago in December in front of a large Christmas window display at Sears filled with Santa and his reindeer and piles of fake snow. In front of him stood a fat two-and-a-half-year-old boy in pleated pants looking like Santa's mini. The fat little boy in the picture was me. I learned growing up that being large does not expand how good you feel or how good you feel about yourself. Feeling bad about myself and being incessantly teased and unable to keep up with the other kids motivated me to learn to watch what I eat, get enough exercise, and control my weight as an adult. While being fat certainly isn't healthy, I can tell you from personal experience, it's also no fun.

According to *Business Insider*, the "average" American woman now wears a size 14 with "plus-sizes, often classified as sizes 14 to 34, needed for 67 percent of the population."[5] If this sounds like you, you are definitely not alone. For many women, this transition to clothes that are several sizes larger begins around menopause. Why is that? Does estrogen influence midlife weight gain in women?

Is Midlife Weight Gain in Women Due to Menopause or Aging?

It is true that the body's metabolism slows down a little each decade, resulting in weight gain of about 1 pound per year due to age.[6, 7] But is your jelly belly a function of weight or weight distribution? Is it just weight gain or has a huge rearrangement of your body's fat seemed to implant a bull's-eye on your belly? And what role do your hormones play?

The transition from your reproductive years to menopause begins when your periods become irregular and ends with your last period.[8] Evidence is mounting that this transition is marked by "unfavorable changes in body composition, abdominal fat deposition and general health outcomes."[9]

Your ethnic group and level of activity should be considered when it comes to obesity and fat distribution.[10] In a study of 16,000 women, telephone interviews were done with US Caucasian, African American, Hispanic, Chinese, and Japanese women.[11] The study concluded that the mean weight of the entire group of women over the 3 years of the study did not differ as the women progressed from premenopause to postmenopause after adjusting for age and other variables. Interestingly, the mean weight of the Caucasian women was significantly greater than the weight of the Chinese women by 2.1 kilograms (about 5 pounds), and the study design led the researchers to determine this increased weight was not due to menopause.

In another study,[12] researchers randomly assigned about 17,000 postmenopausal women who were not using hormone therapy to either a control group that ate whatever it wanted or a different group with a healthier diet that included among other things increased fruits, vegetables, and whole grains. After a year, women in the group who ate a healthy diet had fewer hot flashes and were three times as likely to have lost weight. You can't control your heritage. You can, however, control what you eat. And it does make a difference in your weight.

What Role Do Hormones Play in Menopause Weight Control?

Once the ovaries of mice are removed, studies have shown that they gained weight no matter what they were fed, because of a change in their metabolism.[13] The mice burned fewer calories even though they ate the same diet, and their existing fat cells got larger from storing larger quantities of fat. They developed more belly fat and more inflammation in their bodies, and they became insulin resistant, meaning their pancreas had to produce more insulin to allow the same amount of glucose to enter their cells. Mice that had their ovaries removed also burned fewer calories with exercise and had less energy, so they were less active.[14] When the mice had their ovaries removed and were given the estrogen 17β-estradiol, they had no weight gain, no larger fat cells, no increased belly fat or inflammation, and no insulin resistance.[15] Some animal studies showed that when given estrogen, the mice became full on smaller portions of food.

What about belly fat, estrogen, and women? Abdominal obesity or belly fat is almost double that of general obesity. It's present in 65.5 percent of American women aged 40 to 59 and 73.8 percent of women aged 60 or more.[16] All this starts in perimenopause as estrogen levels begin to decline. The lower estrogen levels appear to cause and to increase the redistribution of fat, making a pear-shaped body into an apple-shaped one. A large number of studies show that postmenopausal women have greater amounts of intra-abdominal fat compared to premenopausal women.[17] A study at the Mayo Clinic[18] helps explain why. The researchers compared fat tissue in pre- and postmenopausal women of similar ages. They found that at the cellular level, the lower levels of estrogen in postmenopausal women caused more activity from two enzymes, adipocyte acyl-CoA synthetase and diacylglycerol acyltransferase, which synthesize and store fat. When estrogen levels were higher in premenopausal women, those enzymes were less active. This is all part of the estrogen fix.

Another recent study drove home the point. A group of researchers at the University of Colorado gave a medication to premenopausal women to temporarily cause menopause. That way, menopausal changes in metabolism due to aging could be eliminated. Once the women were in menopause, the researchers compared the effects of giving half of the participants either estradiol or a placebo.[19] The women who did not take estradiol developed more belly fat and lost bone mass in their spines and hips. There was no change in the women who received estradiol.

So increased fat production and storage is causing waist sizes to get larger, in the form of the "love handles" you can feel and the internal fat you cannot. That is where heart disease, high cholesterol, inflammation, and diabetes risks lie in ambush.

The visceral, or internal, belly fat is more than just an accumulation of jelly belly. Visceral fat is a hormone-making machine that produces unhealthy substances such as adipokines that contribute to insulin resistance, type 2 diabetes, changes in tissue metabolism, and metabolic syndrome.[20]

Risk Factors for Metabolic Syndrome

According to the American Heart Association and the National Heart, Lung, and Blood Institute, you have metabolic syndrome if you have *three* of the five risk factors below:

Large waist size	*For men:* 40 inches or larger *For women:* 35 inches or larger
Cholesterol: high triglycerides	*Either* 150 mg/dL or higher *or* Using a cholesterol medicine
Cholesterol: low good cholesterol (HDL)	*Either* *For men:* Less than 40 mg/dL *For women:* Less than 50 mg/dL *or* Using a cholesterol medicine
High blood pressure	*Either* Having blood pressure of 135/85 mm Hg or greater *or* Using a high blood pressure medicine
Blood sugar: high fasting glucose level	100 mg/dL or higher

Metabolic syndrome increases the risk of stroke, type 2 diabetes, and heart disease. Get a fun and easy way to learn the details of metabolic syndrome from my music video, "Metabolic Syndrome Song." View it at EstrogenFixBook.com/resources.

You don't have to be obese when your estrogen window opens with your last menstrual period[21] to gain more fat in and on your body. By the third year of a study, perimenopausal or postmenopausal women of all ethnic groups who were *not* overweight had more total fat, percentage fat mass, "love handle" fat, and "vicious" fat.[22] Women of Indian origin have an additional significantly increased risk of type 2 diabetes, but it isn't clear if it is due to menopause or other reasons. Chinese women also have an additional independent factor that contributes to belly fat.[23] The take-home message is that with aging comes a slow and steady weight gain you can address with exercise and healthy nutrition. But a large amount of the belly fat of menopause comes from fat finding a new home in your belly, both as "love handles" and as "vicious" fat even if you appear thin. Interestingly, if a woman is overweight during her premenopause years, her cycles tend to be longer and the age of natural menopause tends to be later.[24]

Does Taking EPT or ET Impact Weight and Weight Distribution?

Both animal and human studies on the impact of menopause on weight and weight distribution associate loss of hormones with increased belly fat, loss of energy, reduction in calories burned with exercise, increased inflammation, and higher risk of type 2 diabetes. Does taking EPT reduce the likelihood of those things?

The limited research available today suggests that taking EPT or ET has little impact on weight or BMI.[25] In other words, it neither stops weight gain nor contributes to it. But does taking estrogen have an impact on the distribution of fat and the amount of belly fat? Here the answer is an overwhelming yes! Most, though not all, studies show that estrogen lowers the body's natural tendency to relocate fat to the belly.[26, 27, 28, 29]

In a subset study of the 2002 estrogen plus progestin WHI study, women who had their body composition measured at baseline and then 3 years later and took EPT were significantly better able to maintain their lean body mass and prevent relocation of fat to their bellies.[30]

There are some subtle things to be aware of with regard to taking estrogen. Although this subset WHI study found oral EPT had a favorable impact on belly fat, oral estrogen has been found to be less effective in protecting lean body mass and preventing belly fat than transdermal

THE ESTROGEN FIX

estrogen.[31, 32] These differences appear to be due to the fact that oral estrogen must first pass through the liver; this lowers growth factors (IGF-1 and IGFBP-3), which causes less positive results and increased risk for heart disease.[33] On the other hand, both oral and transdermal estrogen alone and EPT improve insulin's ability to move glucose into cells of the body, which lowers the likelihood of type 2 diabetes.[34] With diabetes on the rise, this is a very important estrogen fix.

Estrogen and Sarcopenic Obesity

Sarcopenia (sar-koe-PEE-nee-uh) is the gradual loss of muscle mass as we age. With menopause, as well, there is a loss of both strength and muscle mass, which creates a number of problems. If you have less core strength, it's harder to avoid falling. If your arms and legs aren't as strong as they once were, it's harder to get up when you do fall. The things that once seemed so easy—lifting children, now grandchildren, or carrying grocery bags—are more difficult and challenging than they were. My friend and colleague Suzanne Andrews, star of the PBS TV show *Functional Fitness with Suzanne Andrews*, tells me that an increasing number of women, as they age, are losing their core strength and compromising their ability to remain independent and vibrant. Menopause and estrogen have a lot to do with sarcopenia and the loss of core strength associated with aging. The good news is that it is preventable.

How does menopause speed up the rate of sarcopenia?[35] Skeletal muscle contains many estrogen receptors, which is how estrogen exerts its influence on muscles. Women who use hormone therapy are about 5 percent stronger than those who don't. This may not seem like much, but considering that women lose about 1 percent of strength per year after menopause and even more after age 70, this added amount of strength could be important in the battle against becoming frail.[36] In addition to estrogen, testosterone has a positive effect on building muscles, which is why so many athletes abuse it. So women who are taking testosterone will also have greater strength as a result,[37] particularly if they have had their ovaries removed and produce lower levels of testosterone.

What happens to sarcopenia if you exercise? In a report of women early in their estrogen window, aged 50 to 57, the volunteers were divided into four groups. The first group was given estrogen plus progestin only. The second group was asked to do high-impact physical exercise. The third group was given a combination of estrogen plus progestin and a high-impact physical exercise proposal. The fourth, or control, group changed nothing for comparison purposes.[38] After the 12 months of the study, high-impact physical exercise alone improved the amount of muscle in the women's legs by 2.2 percent; EPT alone improved muscles 6.3 percent, and when combined with high-impact physical exercise, it improved muscles by 7.1 percent. The ability to jump higher improved in the combined group by 17.2 percent. The control group that neither exercised nor received EPT declined in the amount of leg and thigh muscle by 0.7 percent, and the amount of fat in their muscles increased by 16.6 percent. The exercise-only group had an increase of fat in their legs and thighs of 4.9 percent, and combined exercise and EPT lost 0.6 percent of the fat originally there. In a review article of more than two dozen prior studies,[39] the authors believed that the muscle that was increased was not only larger with exercise plus EPT, but also of higher quality, and that "the specific ovarian hormone important for strength is estradiol." In separate studies,[40, 41] resistance training plus EPT increased strength between 8 and 14 percent.

What does this mean for you? Not exercising and not taking estrogen cause muscle loss and increase fat, making you weaker and heavier. Exercise alone definitely helps prevent this. EPT alone helps prevent it even more, and combining the two keeps you leaner and stronger for longer. That's another important estrogen fix.

I don't want you to think you must take estrogen to control your belly fat. You can still make an impact by eating a healthy diet and exercising regularly.

For example, the Women's Healthy Lifestyle Project[42] studied whether or not lifestyle alone could prevent midlife weight gain. It was a randomized trial that followed 535 premenopausal women aged 44 to 50 through menopause. Roughly half the women were asked to eat a low-calorie diet of about 1,300 calories per day (25 percent total fat, 7 percent saturated fat, 100 mg/day of total cholesterol) and exercise enough to burn an extra 1,000 to 1,500 calories per week. The other half ate their usual diet and went about their usual activities. The goal was to see whether lifestyle changes alone could help women lose between 5 and 15 pounds during the study or at least not gain weight. The women were followed for 5 years. In the end the diet and exercise group lost more inches off their waistlines (on average about 1 inch) and were more likely to have remained at or below their baseline weight. So while weight gain and belly fat are huge midlife issues, they're not a foregone conclusion. We learned that taking estrogen helps make controlling belly fat a little easier. Starting estrogen at the estrogen window prevents the initial muscle and strength loss and the increased accumulation of fat that occurs naturally.

When we combine the information from these studies with the fact that without estrogen women tend to have greater muscle loss, larger amounts of fat, thinner bones, and weight gain with aging, it's clear that unless women eat healthfully, exercise, and possibly use estrogen, the end result is overweight women with sarcopenic obesity. You cannot sit this one out.

The Estrogen Fix and Your Gut

The human microbiome has been receiving a great deal of media attention lately. The microbiome refers to the 3 pounds of bacteria that live in your intestinal tract. They are responsible for everything from digesting food to manufacturing vitamins to brain function, and perhaps even playing a role in obesity, cancer, and other diseases.[43] These 100 trillion good bacteria in our inner ecosystem contain two million unique bacterial genes compared to the mere 23,000 genes in all the cells of our bodies. And these bacteria are active in creating important hormones that influence mood, such as gamma-aminobutyric acid (GABA, which calms anxiety), dopamine, and serotonin. These are the same hormones that were discussed in Chapter 6. In the intestines, they may play an essential role in the "anxious feeling" in your gut that coincides with depression and anxiety. One thing is clear: The gut microbiome is not passive—it interacts with its host, which is you, in many ways and all the time.

I explained in Chapter 8 how estrogen affects the lining of the vagina and the bacteria that live there. Studies are showing that with menopause and less estrogen, there are fewer "good" lactobacillus strains and more vaginal dryness. That negatively affects genes that help the vagina remain strong as a barrier to disease and activates genes associated with inflammation. As mentioned, estrogen plays a major role in the microbiome of the vagina and in vaginal health.

Many things affect which bacteria live in your vagina and gut:

processed foods, healthy foods, antibiotics, stress, probiotics, and medications, such as estrogen. Studies continuously show that which specific bacteria live in your gut determine how effectively you think, behave, feel, remain well, and a whole lot more, while the bacteria living in your vagina determine the health of your vagina.

When I talk about the importance of diet and nutrition in this book, I encourage you to begin thinking about how your diet affects your gut microbiome. I believe one reason women who eat a healthy diet are better able to lose weight is because their food choices create a healthier gut microbiome. As we learn more about the association between a healthy diet and the human microbiome, we will have a better scientific understanding of how your gut microbiome affects estrogen metabolism. We already know that the gut microbiomes of men and women differ, and the most likely reason for that is estrogen[44] and possibly testosterone. When a male's gut microbiome is put under the microscope after castration, it is notably similar to the gut microbiome of a female. Also, in a study[45] 60 healthy postmenopausal women aged 55 to 69 who had not recently used either antibiotics or estrogen had their gut microbiomes tested. The ones with the most diverse gut microbiomes were able to metabolize and excrete more estrogen in their urine than those women with less diverse gut microbiomes. The researchers believe this will put those women at less risk of breast cancer.

Estrogen, particularly oral estrogen, is processed in the liver, and some of it enters the gut. There estrogen interacts with each woman's gut microbiome, and some of these bacteria are able to metabolize estrogen. One enzyme produced by certain bacteria, beta-glucuronidase, is present in the guts of about 44 percent of women with healthy estrogen metabolism.[46] Some people think these bacteria play a regulatory role in how much estrogen is in a woman's bloodstream, and taking antibiotics throws off these bacteria's regulation of estrogen. As this line of thinking and science becomes more established, it may be possible to impact any negative effects of estrogen by giving women probiotics with the "right" kind of bacteria.[47] What it means to me now is to encourage you to do just what your mother said: Eat your fruits and vegetables and unprocessed foods. Limit excess sugar, sodas, and packaged foods. Avoid taking antibiotics unless absolutely necessary. And realize that your intestinal health plays an important role in your overall health, particularly if your estrogen window is open and you are taking estrogen and getting an estrogen fix. In addition, low estrogen levels that occur in menopause lower the nitric oxide levels in your gut just as they do in your blood vessels.[48] The end result is that the intestines slow down, which can cause a negative impact on digestion. All this unbalances the bacteria of your intestinal tract.

Current research says that if your gut bacteria are optimized, more of the estrogen you take will be metabolized and excreted rather than recirculated in your bloodstream. So even though you are taking the same amount of estrogen, your body will have lower exposure to it. That in turn may lower the risk of certain cancers, such as cancer of the uterine lining or breast. Certainly in the short term, it is believed that the health of your gut microbiome contributes to difficulty with weight loss due to increased inflammation. Eating fresh fruits and vegetables, unprocessed foods, and bacteria-boosting fermented foods, such as pickles, kimchi, sauerkraut, and kefir, may actually improve your gut microbiome and help you with weight loss.

Estrogen and Diabetes

I would be remiss as a health-care provider if I didn't mention the effect that America's obesity epidemic is currently having on the number of people diagnosed with type 2 diabetes. According to the American Diabetes Association, in 2012, 29.1 million Americans, or 9.3 percent of the US population, had diabetes, and more than half were women. Of the 29.1 million Americans with diabetes, 21 million were undiagnosed. Currently one-fourth of Americans 65 and older have diabetes. In addition, one in three Americans has prediabetes–their blood sugar is above normal but not high enough to be type 2 diabetes. The good news is that prediabetes is often reversible with increased exercise, better food choices, and weight loss.

In midlife, diabetes is particularly common. As discussed in this chapter, menopause is a time when many women gain weight and experience insulin resistance. Add to this the increase in belly fat and metabolic syndrome and you've got a perfect storm for type 2 diabetes. It's what Dr. Mark Hyman in his book *The Blood Sugar Solution* calls diabesity. By 2020 it will affect one in two Americans, but 90 percent of the people who have it won't be diagnosed. In perimenopause and menopause diabetes is sometimes particularly difficult to diagnose because many of the symptoms are the same:

- Frequent urination
- Night sweats
- Anxiety
- Mood swings
- Foggy thinking
- Dry, itchy skin
- Vaginal infections

At the beginning of this chapter I recalled the story of my youth and how being obese was not a happy time. In a subset of the Nurses' Health Study, women aged 30 to 55 with diabetes were 29 percent more likely to develop depression and were 53 percent more likely to develop depression if they had to take insulin.[49] As I've said throughout this book, menopause and estrogen impact all of you, not just some of you. One of the most positive findings of the WHI study was that taking estrogen plus progestin or estrogen alone lowered the risk of type 2 diabetes. In the EPT arm of the study there was a 21 percent reduction.[50] In the estrogen-only arm, the incidence of diabetes was also less.[51] Estrogen makes insulin more efficient in getting glucose into cells, meaning less insulin resistance and this is another estrogen fix.[52]

Proof of the benefits of estrogen on your risk of diabetes comes from a study by the University of Colorado. The researchers studied type 2 diabetes in postmenopausal women. The women who began estrogen within 6 years of menopause were statistically less likely to develop type 2 diabetes than were the women who began taking estrogen 10 or more years after menopause.[53] Once again, there is an estrogen window that influences your risk for developing type 2 diabetes, just as it does for heart disease, dementia, breast cancer, osteoporosis, and other illnesses.

Keeping Fit, Staying Energized

Having a fit body and maintaining consistent energy levels in midlife isn't easy for all the reasons explained in this chapter. Yes, nature and time are working against you. Weight tends to redistribute itself as belly fat, along with a slow, steady addition of weight each year as you age, if you do nothing. Good eating, exercise, and sleep will help you maintain your weight and fitness level. Creating habits and setting goals you can stick with will allow you to make lifestyle changes. Start by increasing your fresh fruit and vegetable consumption by adding two or three more servings to your daily diet. Walking 10,000 steps a day is fine; you don't have to train for a marathon or an Ironman competition. Add some pickled beets, string beans, cauliflower, or other vegetables to your meals and include a little fermented food. Your gut microbiome will be affected by the food choices you make, and in turn will metabolize any estrogen you take and any already in your body, depending on the composition of your gut bacteria.

Taking estrogen at the opening of your estrogen window will offer the easiest and best solution to controlling an expanding waistline and living a fit and energized life.

FITNESS AND lifestyle consultant and author Kathy Smith has been at the forefront of the fitness and health industry for more than 30 years. Kathy has contributed so much to keeping women healthy and informed about their health, especially through menopause, with her book *Moving Through Menopause*. I interviewed Kathy for her thoughts and tips on staying fit after menopause. (You can read her entire interview and watch her video in issue 25 of HotYearsMag.com.)

DR. MACHE SEIBEL: Women are surprised and frustrated to find that they tend to put on weight around the belly during menopause. What exercises do you suggest to get rid of belly fat?

KATHY SMITH: If your pants are getting tighter and you can't zip them up, it's time to take some action and focus on the different sets of muscles that make up your abdominal core. The rectus abdominis muscles go from the pelvis to the rib cage and are the muscles used in crunches. When you put your hands on your waist and twist from side to side, you're using the transverse abdominis or oblique muscles. To find this muscle, pull your belly button to your spine. The transverse muscles are the ones that need strengthening to keep your tummy from becoming a jelly belly. To strengthen them, pull your belly button into your spine, hold for a count of three, release, and repeat at least 10 times. Do these frequently—while sitting in a chair, standing in line, or just about anywhere—with concentration and focus. If necessary, put your hand on your belly to feel the pull and release.

Planks are one of the best all-around exercises you can do to get rid of belly fat and strengthen your core. In addition, planks are also good for your arms and your legs—two other places where body fat tends to gather as we get older. A plank position is the top of a pushup. If you can't hold the top of a pushup, go down to your elbows. If a pushup is too hard on your hands or your joints, go down to your elbows and get your body straight like an ironing board. Shoulders are down and the ankles, the hips, and the shoulders are all in one straight line. Drop your butt and then use those transverse muscles to your lift your belly and hold the position for 30 seconds. As you learn to engage those muscles, you will be able to hold the pose for 1 minute or more. Do planks daily and you *will* see results.

MS: Taking care of children and parents, working, and running a household all cut into a woman's "me time." Do you have any tips working a fitness regimen into busy lives?

KS: Yes! Even if you can't make it to the gym five times a week, be sure to keep moving throughout the day. Studies show that sitting is the new smoking. That means if you go out for a 30-minute walk in the morning, sit for 8 hours at your office, have dinner, and then watch TV for 3 hours, you're negating that morning walk. Find ways to engage your body throughout the day, parking farther from the grocery store entrance, or walking up a few flights of stairs instead of taking the elevator. Consider purchasing a treadmill desk. Take all phone calls standing up rather than sitting in a chair. Those little things do add up.

After the age of 30, we all begin to lose muscle mass every year. Muscle loss accelerates during perimenopause and menopause, so you have to make sure to do exercises for all the major muscle groups—biceps, triceps, chest, back, butt, hamstrings, and quads. Functional fitness, or functional exercise, refers to movements that use almost all those muscles in one exercise, just as you do in everyday life. Picking up a child. Pulling weeds from the garden. Reaching up for items. Carrying groceries. Do these chores with awareness—pulling in your abdominal muscles and flexing or extending them—and your body will benefit.

MS: *The Estrogen Fix* shows that estrogen has a powerful effect on maintaining strong bones. What else should women focus on when it comes to their bone health?

KS: The best thing you can do to keep from falling and potentially breaking a bone is to work on your balance. I recommend doing static balance as soon as possible. Start with *"I'm standing on one leg, I'm going to lift the other leg up, and I'm going to balance for 10 seconds."* The next time, lift your leg a little bit higher, try closing your eyes, or lift your arms overhead. Then you can repeat this exercise on the other leg.

As we age, think about all the things, from sitting down to getting in and out of a car to opening a jar of pickles, that require strength. I have people start by learning how to do a proper squat. They say, "Oh, I can't squat. My knees are bad." I say, "Every time you sit down to go to the bathroom and you stand back up again, you're doing a squat action." It's essential to learn those movements when you can.

MS: What's the one bit of dietary advice you give to women during menopause?

KS: Eat your greens! We're all told to cut out sugars and processed carbohydrates to avoid metabolic syndrome and belly fat, but what satisfying foods can you replace them with? Greens! Anything green! Every single day make sure you eat some greens—spinach, kale, chard, arugula—whether in a salad, blended into smoothies, or gently steamed, as well as other colorful fruits and vegetables in a rainbow of colors.

Add pickles and other fermented foods to your diet. You always want to make sure that the bacteria in your belly are going to help with digestion and elimination. If you're constipated and not eliminating properly, then you're not going to have a good solid belly, no matter how many exercises you do. Contributing quality bacteria to your microbiome with fermented foods can help maintain gastrointestinal balance.

Often times, people think they're hungry, when they're actually dehydrated. Dehydration can lead to fatigue, headaches, dry skin, constipation, and a host of other ailments. Stay hydrated throughout the day by drinking 8 to 12 glasses of water rather than diet sodas or drinks with sugar.

MS: How can women use exercise to lower stress?

KS: Stress is a fact of modern-day living. It's not going anywhere, and the best chance we have for dealing with it is to alter how we react to stressful situations. For women, putting themselves before caring for others can be difficult and requires effort. By nature, women are nurturers. Double that stress if you're a woman sandwiched between parenting children at home and looking after aging parents or other family members. You'll see an immediate change in your stress levels and moods if you take care of yourself first. Make a real effort to do something nice for yourself every day. Don't skip the gym or your morning walk. Call a friend. Learn to meditate. Turn on some music. Start the day by mentally listing all the people you're grateful for. All of these things create time for exercise and help to lower stress.

Chapter 10

Talking to Your Health-Care Provider about Estrogen and the Estrogen Fix

The Estrogen Fix includes all the information you need to make some important choices that will change your life for the better. Now it's time to put that knowledge to use and take action.

With *The Estrogen Fix,* you now have the most up-to-date information available about estrogen and hormone therapy—as much as many doctors and other health-care providers know. You've learned about the relationship between estrogen and your entire body and the impact that estrogen can have on your brain, breasts, bones, bladder, heart, fitness, weight, skin, vaginal tissues, and more. You understand the important differences between ET and EPT. You know there are differences between oral and other routes of taking estrogen. You know about the different kinds of progestogens. You understand that you have an estrogen window and when your estrogen window opens. You are now in a position to participate in treatment decisions that will impact the rest of your life. You can share what you know with friends and family members who are seeking answers to the same questions. Finally, you are informed and empowered to ask questions and make decisions about taking ET or EPT.

A very powerful transformation has taken place in your life.

With all you've learned, it's now time to make some important decisions. Whether or not to take estrogen is an individual and individualized decision. Since estrogen is a prescription medication, the choice to use it must be made in partnership with your health-care provider. It's time to plan talking with your doctor, nurse, or other provider about estrogen and you. Here are some things to consider as you prepare for that conversation:

- What emotional concerns still remain unanswered?
- What lifestyle behaviors need to change?
- What symptoms or concerns are most worrisome?
- What do you want to tell or ask your health-care provider?
- What other information is needed to thrive beyond menopause in addition to understanding your estrogen window?

In reading *The Estrogen Fix*, you've already taken the first steps on your journey toward creating your own personal menopause breakthrough by deciding whether or not estrogen is right for you. With the knowledge you've gained from reading *The Estrogen Fix,* you can consider your health and personal preferences and optimize your visit with your health-care provider. Just as you prepare for your retirement with financial strategies to make sure you have enough money in the bank to live beyond menopause, you can do proactive things to remain physically and mentally healthy and thrive beyond menopause.

Finding the Right Health-Care Provider

Like any other professionals, health-care providers have their individual opinions, approaches, and treatments for various conditions and illnesses. Finding the right health-care provider includes asking two questions: What do I want to accomplish? And is the provider I'm seeing knowledgeable and flexible enough to help me achieve those goals? When treating the symptoms of menopause, some health-care providers aren't comfortable prescribing either ET or EPT and prefer only alternative or complementary therapies. The reverse is also true. The important thing is to find a provider who is open to your needs and keeps in mind the question I keep coming back to: What do you want to accomplish?

Many health-care providers still aren't aware of the benefits of estrogen, or they may be aware of the benefits but don't realize that the risks of estrogen are much lower if it's taken in your estrogen window. Ask some of them about taking any kind of estrogen and they will quote chapter and verse the findings of the 2002 WHI study, which was based on faulty analysis and limited to information about EPT. Keep asking around for a health-care provider who is knowledgeable in the field of menopause. To find a menopause expert, ask a female friend or relative for a recommendation. Ask your primary-care provider. If you live in the United States or Canada, you can also do a search on the North American Menopause Society's Web site. Physicians and other health-care providers who have passed a competency examination (NAMS Certified Menopause Practitioner) are noted. There are other practitioners who are certainly qualified and experienced and have not taken the NAMS Menopause Practitioner test.

One thing is certain: There's a lot for you to accomplish during a short visit with your provider. You need to update the practitioner on new health habits (good and bad) or health problems; ask important questions; discuss any fears or anxieties; have a thorough exam; and leave with instructions for the next year and appointments for interval follow-up visits. Here are some tips to help you get the most out of a visit with your doctor.

Bring a notebook and/or a friend or a tape recorder. While you think you'll be able to recall everything discussed during your visit, how much will you remember once you leave the office?[1] You may be anxious, embarrassed, half-dressed, coping with brain fog, or all of the above. In doctor appointments that have been recorded, when people are anxious but think they're listening carefully, they forget between 40 and 80 percent of what was said almost immediately,[2] and about half of what they remember is incorrect.[3] It's totally understandable; when you're undressed, nervous, and getting scary or complicated information, it's hard to remember anything.

When you bring a notebook, you can write down everything the provider says, so you can recall the information after your visit. If you have questions, ask for clarifications. People often don't realize they can bring a friend or family member with them. Think how comforting it is to have another set of eyes and ears with you. That person can help make sure you ask all your questions and serve as a second set of ears to remember the answers you may forget. And don't worry if you're going to have a physical examination; they can step behind the curtain or out of the room temporarily so you don't have to worry about being embarrassed. Having another person with you can be very helpful. If you need an interpreter or someone to sign for you, ask. Most hospitals have people available to either come in person or listen in by phone.

Your provider may or may not agree to being recorded. But you can be prepared or ask ahead of time so you don't surprise them, and he or she can let you know their thoughts on taping the conversation. It may also be possible to record a specific set of directions rather than the entire office visit, which may be an acceptable alternative if your health-care provider does object to taping the entire visit.

Write down a list of questions. Do you have any specific worries? Do you have any physical or emotional problems you really want to discuss? Are there questions that are difficult for you to remember or difficult for you to discuss? Is there a part of your medical history or family history that requires a detailed explanation? Write down your questions so you don't forget to ask them.

Keep a symptoms diary. In the weeks or months ahead of your visit, keeping a diary of your symptoms can make certain you don't forget issues that should be discussed at your visit. Examples might be the frequency of hot flashes, pressure on your chest, palpitations, difficulty focusing, shortness of breath, vaginal dryness, and others. Go to EstrogenFixBook.com/resources for the menopause symptom checklist you can use for your visit.

Book enough time. Most office visits are about 15 minutes, while some are even shorter. That is not enough time to discuss your estrogen fix. Make sure your health-care provider knows you are there for this discussion and gives you the necessary time to answer your questions. If for some reason all your questions aren't answered, book a follow-up appointment before you leave the office.

The Pelvic Exam

Nobody looks forward to a pelvic exam. While they can be uncomfortable and some health-care providers are gentler than others, a regular pelvic exam is essential whether or not you decide to take estrogen. The recommendations for how often to get a pelvic exam from a gynecologist, skilled internist, nurse, or family practitioner along with a Pap test to check for cancer of the cervix (opening of the uterus) have undergone some changes. A Pap test can be done less often if you have no pelvic symptoms and have had three normal Pap tests in a row and no abnormal results in the past 10 years. Thus far studies have not shown that getting an ultrasound of the ovaries to look for ovarian cancer saves lives. But with less-frequent pelvic exams now becoming the norm, yearly pelvic exams and pelvic ultrasounds should be considered if there is a family history of ovarian cancer. Although several studies suggest that pelvic ultrasounds are not cost-effective for diagnosing ovarian cancer, I recommend having a discussion with your health-care provider about an ultrasound of the ovaries if you have a family history of breast cancer, because there can be a genetic link between breast cancer and ovarian cancer. You may also want to ask about seeing a genetic counselor. Pelvic ultrasounds also assess the thickness of the uterine lining and "see" the other pelvic anatomy. I think pelvic ultrasounds are particularly important if a gynecological practitioner doesn't perform your pelvic exam. Most internists and family medicine practitioners are not as experienced with pelvic exams as gynecologists.

For women who are not sexually active or who have genitourinary syndrome of menopause, a vaginal exam can be particularly uncomfortable. There are speculums designed for just this purpose—smaller than the ones typically used. For a few of my patients, I use a smaller pediatric speculum. The shape of the speculum matters too. Graves speculums are wider and Pederson speculums are narrower and more comfortable, even for women who don't have genitourinary syndrome of menopause. Warming the speculums ahead of time also adds to their comfort. Your health-care provider can run warm (not hot) water over the speculum before an exam if he or she doesn't have a warmer for them. The water can often serve as the lubricant to avoid the messiness of a gel. Most women don't like plastic speculums because they are larger than necessary and open wider than metal ones. If you have any choice in the matter, say no to plastic speculums.

If you are about to begin taking estrogen, your health-care provider may ask you to have either an endometrial biopsy of the uterine lining to be sure the uterine lining is normal and has no precancerous changes, or a pelvic ultrasound to determine the thickness of the uterine lining. If the lining is 4.4 millimeters or less thick, there is virtually no risk of abnormal cell types.[4, 5] When the lining is 4.5 millimeters or greater, an endometrial biopsy is needed to be sure no cancer or precancer is present. The Pap test does not test for endometrial cancer, though rarely it may provide a diagnosis. Ultrasound can also determine if there is a polyp in the uterine lining or other structural abnormalities that might need to be addressed.

In 2012 the American College of Obstetricians and Gynecologists with support from the American Cancer Society recommended that most women only need a Pap test to screen for cervical cancer every 3 to 5 years rather than annually. As a result, I've found that many women think they don't need an annual pelvic exam, which couldn't be further from the truth. A pelvic examination is the first step in determining if there are problems in the vagina and uterus. If there is any indication of an abnormality, further tests such as an ultrasound or an endometrial biopsy can then be ordered. The annual exam is an opportunity to examine the breasts, ovaries, and uterus and ask important screening questions about how you are doing if you're taking estrogen or other medications, and many other things about your health, wellness, and relationships. Don't give up your annual pelvic examination.

The Breast Exam

During your visit your doctor will likely do a breast exam to notice if there are any discharges from the nipples, lumps or dimples in the skin of the breast, or any other abnormalities. I recommend doing a breast self-examination at the same time of every month if you are still having periods or taking HT. That way you can point your doctor to any suspicions or worries or changes you might have noticed. I know many women who have discovered suspicious lumps on their breasts and saved valuable time because they were able to alert their doctors. If you're unsure how to do a breast self-exam, this visit is a good time to ask how.

What Other Tests Should I Consider?

Your health should be about looking at the body as a whole. While baseline and annual mammograms and bone density tests are essential, knowing that other organs of your body are healthy is just as important, because they may reveal treatable conditions and diseases. For example, an eye examination may raise concerns about glaucoma, retinal issues, or dry eyes, and it can also indicate arterial problems in other parts of your body as well as your eyes. Your teeth and gums should be checked twice a year. Teeth are bones, and tooth loss or problems with your teeth and gums may indicate osteoporosis.[6] Gums may harbor bacteria that can be a source of infections.

When blood is taken to check your cholesterol numbers, your vitamin D levels should be checked as well. Low levels of 25-hydroxy vitamin D, which are present in up to 75 percent of women in menopause, have been associated with an increased chance of developing breast and pancreatic cancers.[7] Low vitamin D levels are also linked to osteoporosis, hot flashes, and mood swings.

I discuss these and other issues when I speak to women's groups or corporations.

Your Estrogen Window of Opportunity for an Estrogen Fix

The Estrogen Fix is a discovery of the information you need to make one of the most important decisions in your life. Is hormone therapy right for you? Now you know that you have a limited window of time to make your decision and implement your choice. You can sit down with your health-care provider as an empowered member of the team helping to frame your own care. You are in an incredibly powerful position.

You can go to your health-care provider's office armed with the confidence and the wisdom you now possess to discuss your options: what dose, which type, when to start, and when to stop. If you choose not to take estrogen, there are good estrogen alternatives. Whatever you choose, you now have the information you need to get the conversation started and make decisions for the right reasons.

Keep in mind that you may be discussing two different approaches to your estrogen fix. If you have a uterus, you will be talking about EPT. If your uterus has been removed, you will be talking about ET. I've mentioned repeatedly throughout *The Estrogen Fix* that these situations require two very different treatments.

Your estrogen window will open at the beginning of menopause and will stay open for approximately 10 years, but certain parts of the body have their own time frames, which vary slightly. For example, the estrogen window for bones is approximately 3 years if you want to regain any lost bone, and up to 6 years if you want to prevent losing even more; the estrogen window for the vagina in general stays open.

If you are taking estrogen alone (ET), the medical consensus is that you can likely take estrogen for 5 years, have a discussion with your doctor, and continue for an additional 5 years. Most women will be able to continue estrogen for the entire 10 years from the start. While a consensus has not been reached, the preliminary information available about the estrogen window for ET suggests that it remains open for even much longer. This is why ongoing discussions with your health-care provider are essential. You can also get updates at DrMache.com.

If you are taking EPT, your estrogen window will again open at the beginning of menopause and continue for 5 years with the opportunity to continue it for an additional 5 years. Using bioidentical progesterone or some of the other approaches I have discussed will most likely expand your estrogen window and allow for much safer use than combining estrogen with Provera. I've also mentioned several very large studies that found low dose estradiol safer for longer than 10 years. EPT is not as straightforward as ET and requires more individualized discussion.

I asked you at the beginning of *The Estrogen Fix,* "How do you feel about estrogen?" That and the other questions at the beginning of this book may have caused you anxiety but can now be asked and answered with confidence. With at least one-third of your life still ahead of you, menopause is the right time to be proactive and preventive for emotional and physical health and wellness in the coming years.

Throughout *The Estrogen Fix,* I've stressed that hormone therapy is just one aspect of optimal health that women should consider. Whether or not you choose to take estrogen and use your estrogen window, you can take other steps—plenty of exercise, good nutrition, quality sleep, and low stress levels—to make sure you remain at the top of your game. The goal is for you to stay well; not get sick and then get well.

Not every decision about your health will be easy or 100 percent clear. You will sometimes have to ask, "How do I want to care for the sum of me, not just some of me?" It's important to use this questioning approach when dealing with your overall *physical* health and well-being: Ask yourself, what do I want to accomplish physically, emotionally, and mentally for a healthy future? It is important to have an action plan that encompasses mind, body, and spirit. Make a commitment to yourself to make that happen!

So What Do I Do Now?

What do you do now? Where do you begin?

You've gotten a lot of information in this book that can dramatically change your life. But for change to be lasting, you have to use this information. I know you've been through a lot, and I respect the fact that you are taking time to get important questions answered. I know that in addition to helping yourself, you will also be a messenger and tell your friends and family about the information you gained. It's time to take action on what you've learned.

Throughout this book, I've talked about making a menopause breakthrough. What do I mean by that? It's a course of action that enables you to improve your mind, body, and spirit.

How do you do that?

I created a free online quiz to help you know where you are in your menopause journey. You can find that free 2-minute quiz at Menopause-Quiz.com. The quiz will help you discover what areas of menopause create the largest challenges for you and how your experience compares with those of other women. After you complete the menopause quiz, you will instantly receive your score and some useful follow up tips to help you as you travel into, through, and beyond menopause.

Learn more about the MenopauseQuiz.com at the end of the book on page 238. Be sure to visit EstrogenFixBook.com and click on "FREE BOOK BONUSES" to receive several valuable gifts. If you have questions, I make a Facebook LIVE "HouseCall" every week. Just visit Ask-DrMache.com to submit your questions in advance and get a link to the **Facebook LIVE Q** & A.

Acknowledgments

Writing *The Estrogen Fix* has required the unraveling of misinformation from the past several decades and then explaining the most recent data and knowledge in a clear and accurate way so everyone can understand estrogen. Doing so required the help and input of a number of people.

I would first like to thank the hundreds of scientists and clinicians who have worked on this topic for sharing their knowledge with me, in particular Dr. Phil Sarrel, who read every word and every footnote of this book and shared his thoughts and input over many conversations. Thank you also to Drs. Mary Jane Minkin and Wulf Utian for their feedback and suggestions on the manuscript. I would also like to thank the North American Menopause Society for its ongoing commitment to clarifying this information. In particular I would like to thank past presidents Drs. Pauline Maki, JoAnn V. Pinkerton, now executive director, and JoAnn E. Manson, one of the lead investigators on the Women's Health Initiative. I also spoke with and interviewed countless other leaders in women's health and in the field of menopause as editor of *The Hot Years-My Menopause Magazine* and incorporated their input.

Thank you also to women's health leaders from various lay organizations who provided their perspectives, including Karen Giblin of Red Hot Mamas, Michelle Robson of EmpowHer, and Sandra Yancey of eWomenNetwork. Each provided perspectives that were incorporated to make certain that this book best served the women it was written for.

I would also like to thank Mary Ann Naples of Rodale for her initial interest in the book, JJ Virgin for her thoughts on how to make it most impactful, my literary agent Coleen O'Shea, who found the perfect home for my book, and Harriet Bell for her help with the manuscript. Thank you also to Jennifer Levesque and the Rodale team for their support of *The Estrogen Fix*. They all shared my vision for getting rid of the fear and uncertainty surrounding estrogen and, instead, for providing women with the most up-to-date information, so they can make informed choices to achieve the healthy and vibrant lives they deserve.

Endnotes

Chapter 1: Estrogen: Behind the Headlines

1   E. Roehm, "A Reappraisal of Women's Health Initiative Estrogen-Alone Trial: Long-Term Outcomes in Women 50–59 Years of Age," *Obstetrics and Gynecology International* (2015): 713295.

2   A. Z. LaCroix et al., "Health Outcomes after Stopping Conjugated Equine Estrogens among Postmenopausal Women with Prior Hysterectomy," *JAMA* 305, no. 13 (2011): 1305–14.

3   N. C. Hazra et al., "Differences in Health at Age 100 According to Sex: Population-Based Cohort Study of Centenarians Using Electronic Health Records," *Journal of the American Geriatrics Society* 63, no. 7 (July 2015): 1331–37.

4   D. M. Herrington, "Hormone Replacement Therapy and Heart Disease: Replacing Dogma with Data," *Circulation* 107 (2003): 2–4.

5   H. K. Ziel and W. D. Finkle, "Increased Risk of Endometrial Carcinoma among Users of Conjugated Estrogens," *New England Journal of Medicine* 293, no. 23 (December 4, 1974): 1167–70.

6   D. C. Smith et al., "Association of Exogenous Estrogen and Endometrial Carcinoma," *New England Journal of Medicine* 293, no. 23 (December 4, 1975): 1164–67.

7   T. M. Mack et al., "Estrogens and Endometrial Cancer in a Retirement Community," *New England Journal of Medicine* 294 (June 3, 1976): 1262–67.

8   V. T. Miller et al., "Effects of Estrogen or Estrogen/Progestin Regimens on Heart Disease Risk Factors in Postmenopausal Women," *JAMA* 273, no. 3 (1995): 199–208.

9   W. Utian, "Hormones after Age 65 Are OK for Some Women," *MenoPause* (blog), June 3, 2015, menopause.org/for-women/menopause-take-time-to-think-about-it/consumers/2015/06/03/hormones-after-age-65-are-ok-for-some-women.

10   Lila O'Connor, ed., "NAMS 2016 Hormone Therapy Position Statement," *OBG Management* 28, no. 10 (October 2016).

Chapter 2: Estrogen and You

1   G. D. Mishra et al., "Early Life Circumstances and Their Impact on Menarche and Menopause," *Women's Health* 5, no. 2 (2009): 175–90.

2   J. L. Kelsey and L. Bernstein, "Epidemiology and Prevention of Breast Cancer," *Annual Review of Public Health* 17 (May 1996): 47–67.

3   "Endometrial Cancer Prevention–For Health Professionals (PDQ): Who Is at Risk?" National Cancer Institute, last modified January 30, 2015, cancer.gov/types/uterine/hp/endometrial-prevention-pdq.

4   S. D. Harlow et al., "Executive Summary of the Stages of Reproductive Aging Workshop + 10: Addressing the Unfinished Agenda of Staging Reproductive Aging," *Menopause* 19, no. 4 (2012): 1–9.

5   Ibid.

6   E. W. Freeman et al., "Anti-Mullerian Hormone as a Predictor of Time to Menopause in Late Reproductive Age Women," *Journal of Clinical Endocrinology & Metabolism* 97, no. 5 (May 2012): 1673–80.

7   N. Siddle, P. Sarrel, and M. Whitehead, "The Effect of Hysterectomy on the Age at Ovarian Failure: Identification of a Subgroup of Women with Premature Loss of Ovarian Function and Literature Review," *Fertility and Sterility* 47, no. 1 (January 1987): 94–100.

8   P. O. Janson and I. Jansson, "The Acute Effect of Hysterectomy on Ovarian Blood Flow," *American Journal of Obstetrics & Gynecology* 127, no. 4 (February 15, 1977): 349–52.

9   C. M. Farquhar et al., "The Association of Hysterectomy and Menopause: A Prospective Cohort Study," *BJOG: An International Journal of Obstetrics and Gynaecology* 112, no. 7 (July 2005): 956–62.

10   A. Z. Souza et al., "Ovarian Histology and Function after Total Abdominal Hysterectomy," *Obstetrics & Gynecology* 68, no. 6 (December 1986): 847–49.

11   Siddle, Sarrel, and Whitehead, "The Effect of Hysterectomy," 94–100.

12   The American Congress of Obstetricians and Gynecologists, *2011 Women's Health Stats & Facts*, accessed October 19, 2015, acog.org/-/media/NewsRoom/MediaKit.pdf.

13   P. Gartoulla et al., "Moderate to Severe Vasomotor and Sexual Symptoms Remain Problematic for Women Aged 60 to 65 Years," *Menopause* 22, no. 7 (2015): 694–701.

14   T. S. Mikkola, H. Savolainen-Peltonen, P. Tuomikoski, et al., "Reduced Risk of Breast Cancer Mortality in Women Using Postmenopausal Hormone Therapy: A Finnish Nationwide-Comparative Study," *Menopause* 23, no. 11 (November 2016): 1199–1203.

15   S. L. Crawford, "What Should Women Expect after Stopping Hormone Therapy?" *Menopause* 4, no. 22 (2015): 367–68.

16   L. Lindh-Astrand et al., "A Randomized Controlled Study of Taper-Down or Abrupt Discontinuation of Hormone Therapy in Women Treated for Vasomotor Symptoms," *Menopause* 17, no. 1 (January–February 2010): 72–79.

17   R. G. Mishra et al., "Medroxyprogesterone Acetate and Dihydrotestosterone Induce Coronary Hyperreactivity in Intact Male Rhesus Monkeys," *Journal of Clinical Endocrinology & Metabolism* 90, no. 6 (June 2005): 3706–14.

18   P. M. Sarrel, "The Differential Effects of Oestrogens and Progestins on Vascular Tone," *Human Reproduction Update* 5, no. 3 (May-June, 1999): 205–9.

19   R. Lobo, "Reproductive Endocrinology: Don't Be So Quick to Stop Hormone-Replacement Therapy," *Nature Reviews Endocrinology* 12, no. 1 (January 2016): 11–13.

Chapter 3: Your Estrogen Fix: Choosing the Right Hormone Therapy for You

1   W. H. Parker et al., "Long-Term Mortality Associated with Oophorectomy Compared with Ovarian Conservation in the Nurses' Health Study," *Obstetrics & Gynecology* 121, no. 4 (April 2013): 709–16.

2   L. T. Shuster et al., "Prophylactic Oophorectomy in Pre-Menopausal Women and Long Term Health–A Review," *Menopause* 14, no. 3 (2008): 111–16.

3   M. Brooks, "Early Surgical Menopause Linked to Early Cognitive Decline," *Medscape Medical News,* January 15, 2013.

4   I. Le Ray, S. Dell'Aniello, F. Bonnetain, et al., "Local Estrogen Therapy and Risk of Breast Cancer Recurrence Among Hormone-Treated Patients: A Nested Case-Control Study," *Breast Cancer Research and Treatment* 135, no. 2 (September 2012): 603–9.

5   J. E. Manson et al., "Menopausal Hormone Therapy and Health Outcomes during the Intervention and Extended Poststopping Phases of the Women's Health Initiative Randomized Trials," *JAMA* 310, no. 13 (October 2, 2013): 1353–68.

6   W. Y. Chen et al., "Moderate Alcohol Consumption during Adult Life, Drinking Patterns, and Breast Cancer Risk," *JAMA* 306 (2011): 1884–90.

7   T. S. Mikkola, H. Savolainen-Peltonen, P. Tuomikoski, et al., "Reduced Risk of Breast Cancer Mortality in Women Using Postmenopausal Hormone Therapy: A Finnish Nationwide Comparative Study," *Menopause* 23, no. 11 (November 2016): 1199–1203.

8   T. J. de Villiers et al., "Global Consensus Statement on Menopausal Hormone Therapy," *Climacteric* 16 (2013): 203–4.

9   M. Canonico et al., "Hormone Therapy and Venous Thromboembolism among Postmenopausal Women: Impact of the Route of Estrogen Administration and Progestogens: The ESTHER Study," *Circulation* 115, no. 7 (February 20, 2007): 840–45.

10   S. Sweetland et al., "Venous Thromboembolism Risk in Relation to Use of Different Types of Postmenopausal Hormone Therapy in a Large Prospective Study," *Journal of Thrombosis and Haemostasis* 10, no. 11 (November 2012): 2277–86.

11   W. A. Rocca et al., "Long-Term Risk of Depressive and Anxiety Symptoms after Early Bilateral Oophorectomy," *Menopause* 15, no. 6 (November–December 2008): 1050–59.

12   W. A. Rocca et al., "Increased Risk of Cognitive Impairment or Dementia in Women Who Underwent Oophorectomy before Menopause," *Neurology* 69, no. 11 (September 11, 2007): 1074–83.

13   P. P. Zandi et al., "Hormone Replacement Therapy and Incidence of Alzheimer Disease in Older Women," *JAMA* 288, no. 17 (2002): 2123-29.

14   W. Xu et al., "Meta-Analysis of Modifiable Risk Factors for Alzheimer's Disease," *Journal of Neurology, Neurosurgery & Psychiatry* (2015).

15   M. A. Fischer et al., "Primary Medication Non-Adherence: Analysis of 195,930 Electronic Prescriptions," *Journal of General Internal Medicine* 25 (2010): 284–90.

16   V. A. Ravnikar, "Compliance with Hormone Therapy," *American Journal of Obstetrics and Gynecology* 156, no. 5 (May 1987): 1332–34.

17   "Female Sexual Dysfunction," WebMD, accessed September 24, 2015, webmd.com/women/guide/sexual-dysfunction-women.

18   E. O. Laumann, A. Paik, and R. C. Rosen, "Sexual Dysfunction in the United States: Prevalence and Predictors," *JAMA* 281, no. 6 (1999): 537–44.

19   M. Robson et al., "Quality of Life in Women at Risk for Ovarian Cancer Who Have Undergone Risk-Reducing Oophorectomy," *Gynecologic Oncology* 89, no. 2 (May 2003): 281–87.

20   N. A. Phillips, "Female Sexual Dysfunction: Evaluation and Treatment," *American Family Physician* 62, no. 1 (July 1, 2000): 127–36.

21   M. H. Beers et al., "Explicit Criteria for Determining Inappropriate Medication Use in Nursing Home Residents," *Archives of Internal Medicine* 151 (1991): 1825–32.

22   Lila O'Connor, ed., "NAMS 2016 Hormone Therapy Position Statement," *OBG Management* 28, no. 10 (October 2016).

23   P. Gartoulla et al., "Moderate to Severe Vasomotor and Sexual Symptoms Remain Problematic for Women Aged 60–65 Years," *Menopause* 22 (2015): 694–701.

24   M. A. Clark et al., *Pharmacology* (Philadelphia: Lippincott Williams & Wilkins, December 2011): 322.

25   N. L. Smith et al., "Lower Risk of Cardiovascular Events in Postmenopausal Women Taking Oral Estradiol Compared with Oral Conjugated Equine Estrogens," *JAMA Internal Medicine* 174, no. 1 (2014): 25–34.

26   T. Parker-Pope, "When Hormone Creams Expose Others to Risks," *New York Times,* October 26, 2010, well.blogs.nytimes.com/2010/10/25/when-hormone-creams-expose-others-to-risks/?_r=0.

27   A. Weissmannn-Brenner, T. Bayevsky, and I. Yoles, "Compliance to Vaginal Treatment–Tablets Versus Cream: A Retrospective 9 Years," *Menopause* 24, no. 1 (January 2017): 73–76.

28   B. R. Bhavnani and F. Z. Stanczyk, "Misconceptions and Concerns about Bioidentical Hormones Used for Custom-Compounded Hormone Therapy," *Journal of Clinical Endocrinology & Metabolism* 97, no. 3 (March 2012): 756–59.

29   www.fda.gov/ForConsumers/ConsumerUpdates/ucm049311.htm.

30   "Compounding Quality Act: Title I of the Drug Quality and Security Act of 2013," US Food and Drug Administration, last modified October 6, 2015, www.fda.gov/Drugs/GuidanceComplianceRegulatoryInformation/Pharmacy Compounding/ucm339764.htm.

31   M. L. Gass, C. A. Stuenkel et al., "Use of Compounded Hormone Therapy in the United States: Report of the North American Menopause Society Survey," *Menopause* 22, no. 12 (December 2015): 1276–84.

32   The North American Menopause Society, "More Women Now Using Compounded Hormones without Understanding the Risks," February 19, 2015, http://www.menopause.org/docs/default-source/2015/cbht-use-trends-gaps.pdf.

33   N. Santoro, G. D. Braunstein, C. L. Butts, et al., "Compounded Bioidentical Hormones in Endocrinology Practice: An Endocrine Society Scientific Statement," *The Journal of Clinical Endocrinology & Metabolism* 101, no. 4 (April 2016): 1318–43.

34   J. E. Manson et al., "Algorithm and Mobile App for Menopausal Symptom Management and Hormonal/Non-Hormonal Therapy Decision Making: A Clinical Decision-Support Tool from the North American Menopause Society," *Menopause* 22, no. 3 (March 2015): 247–53.

35   T. S. Mikkola et al., "Estradiol-Based Postmenopausal Hormone Therapy and Risk of Cardiovascular and All-Cause Mortality," *Menopause* 22, no. 9 (September 2015): 976–83.

36   "WHI Study Finds No Heart Disease Benefit, Increased Stroke Risk with Estrogen Alone," National Institutes of Health, April 13, 2004, www.nhlbi.nih.gov/news/press-releases/2004/whi-study-finds-no-heart -disease-benefit-increased-stroke-risk-with-estrogen-alone.

37   "NHLBI Advisory for Physicians on the WHI Trial of Conjugated Equine Estrogens Versus Placebo," National Institutes of Health, accessed September 25, 2015, www.nhlbi.nih.gov/whi/e-a_advisory.htm.

38   North American Menopause Society, "Role of Progestogen in Hormone Therapy for Postmenopausal Women: Position Statement of The North American Menopause Society," *Menopause* 10, no. 2 (March–April 2003): 113–32.

39   T. S. Mikkola, P. Tuomikoski, H. Lyytinen, et al., "Estradiol-Based Postmenopausal Hormone Therapy and Risk of Cardiovascular and All-Cause Mortality," *Menopause* 22, no. 9 (September 2015): 976–83.

40   C. Campagnoli et al., "Progestins and Progesterone in Hormone Replacement Therapy and the Risk of Breast Cancer," *Journal of Steroid Biochemistry and Molecular Biology* 96, no. 2 (July 2005): 95–108.

41   Ibid.

42   C. E. Wood et al., "Effects of Estradiol with Micronized Progesterone or Medroxyprogesterone Acetate on Risk Markers for Breast Cancer in Postmenopausal Monkeys," *Breast Cancer Research and Treatment* 101, no. 2 (January 2007): 125–34.

43   A. Fournier et al., "Breast Cancer Risk in Relation to Different Types of Hormone Replacement Therapy in the E3n-Epic Cohort," *International Journal of Cancer* 114, no. 3 (April 10, 2005): 448–54.

44   B. Ettinger, A. Pressman, and A. Van Gessel, "Low-Dosage Esterified Estrogens Opposed by Progestin at 6-Month Intervals," *Obstetrics & Gynecology* 98, no. 2 (August 2001): 205–11.

45   S. Palacios et al., "A 7-Year Randomized, Placebo-Controlled Trial Assessing the Long-Term Efficacy and Safety of Bazedoxifene in Postmenopausal Women with Osteoporosis: Effects on Bone Density and Fracture," *Menopause* 22 (2015): 806–13.

46 P .V. Pinkerton, J. A. Harvey, K. Pan et al., "Breast Effect of Bazedoxifene-Conjugated Estrogen: A Randomized Controlled Trial," *Obstetrics & Gynecology* 121, no. 5 (2013): 959–68.

47 R. Kegan, B. S. Komm, K. A. Ryan, et al., "Timing and Persistence of Effect of Conjugated Estrogen/Gazedoxifene in Postmenopausal Women," *Menopause* 23, no. 11 (November 2016): 1204–13.

48 de Villiers et al., "Global Consensus Statement," 203–4.

49 W. Wuttke, Ch. Gorkow, and H. Jarry, "Dopaminergic Compounds in *Vitex Agnus Castus*," in *Phytopharmaka in Forschung und klinischer Anwendung*, ed. D. Loew and N. Rietbrock (Dresden, Germany: Steinkopff Verlag Dopaminergic, 1995), 81–91.

50 J. D. Hirata et al., "Does Dong Quai Have Estrogenic Effects in Postmenopausal Women? A Double-Blind, Placebo-Controlled Trial," *Fertility and Sterility* 68 (1997): 981–86.

51 R. Chenoy et al., "Effect of Oral Gamolenic Acid from Evening Primrose Oil on Menopausal Flushing," *British Medical Journal* 308 (1994): 501–3.

52 R. J. Baber et al., "Randomized Placebo-Controlled Trial of an Isoflavone Supplement and Menopausal Symptoms in Women," *Climacteric* 2, no. 2 (June 1999): 85–92.

53 L. B. Nachtigall et al., "The Effects of Isoflavones Derived from Red Clover on Vasomotor Symptoms and Endometrial Thickness" (presented at the 9th International Menopause Society World Congress on the Menopause, Yokohama, Japan, October 17–21, 1999).

54 P. F. Cheng et al., "Do Soy Isoflavones Improve Cognitive Function in Postmenopausal Women? A Meta-Analysis," *Menopause* 22 (July 2015): 198–206.

55 M. Messina and C. Gleason, "Evaluation of the Potential Antidepressant Effects of Soybean Isoflavones," *Menopause* 23, no. 12 (December 2016): 1348–60.

56 S. J. Nechuta et al., "Soy Food Intake after Diagnosis of Breast Cancer and Survival: An In-Depth Analysis of Combined Evidence from Cohort Studies of US and Chinese Women," *American Journal of Clinical Nutrition* 96 (2012): 123–32.

57 M. Messina et al., "It's Time for Clinicians to Reconsider Their Proscription against the Use of Soyfoods by Breast Cancer Patients," *Oncology* 27, no. 5 (May 2013): 430–37.

58 The North American Menopause Society, "The Role of Soy Isoflavones in Menopausal Health: Report of The North American Menopause Society/Wulf H. Utian Translational Science Symposium in Chicago, IL (October 2010)," *Menopause* 18, no. 7 (July 2011): 732–53.

59 L. Nachtigall, "Comparative Study: Replens versus Local Estrogen in Menopausal Women," *Fertility and Sterility* 61 (1994): 178–80.

60 H. Y. Chiu et al., "Effects of Acupuncture on Menopause-Related Symptoms and Quality of Life in Women in Natural Menopause: A Meta-Analysis of Randomized Controlled Trials," *Menopause* 22 (July 2015): 234–44.

61   S. M. Green et al., "Cognitive-Behavioral Group Treatment for Menopausal Symptoms: A Pilot Study," *Archives of Women's Mental Health* 16, no. 4 (August 2013): 325–32.

62   D. F. Archer et al., "Effects of Ospemifene on the Female Reproductive and Urinary Tracts: Translation from Preclinical Models into Clinical Evidence," *Menopause* 22 (July 2015): 786–99.

63   F. Labrie et al., "Efficacy of Intravaginal Dehydroepiandrosterone (DHEA) on Moderate to Severe Dyspareunia and Vaginal Dryness, Symptoms of Vulvovaginal Atrophy, and of the Genitourinary Syndrome of Menopause," *Menopause* 23, no. 3, (March 2016): 243–56.

Chapter 4: The Estrogen Fix and Your Breasts

1   K. D. Kochanek et al., "Deaths: Final Data for 2009," *National Vital Statistics Reports* 60, no. 3 (December 29, 2011).

2   A. M. Kaunitz and J. E. Manson, "Failure to Treat Menopausal Symptoms: A Disconnect between Clinical Practice and Scientific Data," *Menopause* 22 (2015): 687–88.

3   A. M. Kaunitz, "Disparity in Menopausal Hormone Therapy Use between Women Obstetrician Gynecologists and Women Overall: Are Obstetrician Gynecologists Underserving Their Patients?" *Menopause* 19 (2012): 1070–71.

4   Kaunitz and Manson, "Failure to Treat Menopausal Symptoms," 687–88.

5   A. M. Kaunitz, "Hormone Therapy and Breast Cancer Risk: Trumping Fear with Facts," *Menopause* 13 (2006): 160–63.

6   R. T. Chlebowski and G. L. Anderson, "Changing Concepts: Menopausal Hormone Therapy and Breast Cancer," *Journal of the National Cancer Institute* 104, no. 7 (2012): 517–27.

7   Chlebowski and Anderson, "Changing Concepts," 517–27.

8   Ibid.

9   J. E. Manson et al., "Menopausal Hormone Therapy and Health Outcomes During the Intervention and Extended Poststopping Phases of the Women's Health Initiative Randomized Trials," *JAMA* 310 (2013): 1353–68.

10   G. L. Anderson et al., "Prior Hormone Therapy and Breast Cancer Risk in the Women's Health Initiative Randomized Trial of Estrogen Plus Progestin," *Maturitas* 55, no. 2 (September 2006): 103–15.

11   T. S. Mikkola, H. Savolainen-Peltonen, P. Tuomikoski, et al., "Reduced Risk of Breast Cancer Mortality in Women Using Postmenopausal Hormone Therapy: A Finnish Nationwide Comparative Study," *Menopause* 23, no. 11 (November 2016): 1199–1203.

12   J. E. Manson et al., "Why the Product Labeling for Low-Dose Vaginal Estrogen Should Be Changed," *Menopause* 21 (2014): 911–16.

13   P. E. Lønning et al., "High-Dose Estrogen Treatment in Postmenopausal Breast Cancer Patients Heavily Exposed to Endocrine Therapy," *Breast Cancer Research Treatment* 67, no. 2 (May 2001): 111–16.

14   "Estrogen and Breast Cancer and Duavee: Dr. Seibel Interview Richard Santen, MD," YouTube video, 7:58, posted by Mache Seibel, March 23, 2014, youtube.com/watch?v=7i8z-Mom03M.

15   J. Russo and I. H. Russo, "DNA Labeling Index and Structure of the Rat Mammary Gland as Determinants of Its Susceptibility to Carcinogenesis," *Journal of the National Cancer Institute* 61 (1978): 1451–59.

16   I. H. Russo, M. Koszalka, and J. Russo, "Effect of Human Chorionic Gonadotropins on Mammary Gland Differentiation and Carcinogenesis," *Carcinogenesis* 11 (1990): 1849–55.

17   P. A. Carney et al., "Individual and Combined Effects of Age, Breast Density, and Hormone Replacement Therapy Use on the Accuracy of Screening Mammography," *Annals of Internal Medicine* 138 (February 4, 2003): 168–75.

18   "Hormone Replacement Therapy and Mammogram Accuracy," ObGyn.net, July 28, 2011, www.obgyn.net/menopause/hormone-replacement-therapy -and-mammogram-accuracy.

19   Ibid.

20   Carney et al., "Individual and Combined Effects," 168–75.

21   P. C. Stomper et al., "Analysis of Parenchymal Density on Mammograms in 1353 Women 25–79 Years Old," *American Journal of Roentgenology* 167 (1996): 1261–65.

22   I. Persson, E. Thurfjell, and L. Holmberg, "Effect of Estrogen and Estrogen-Progestin Replacement Regimens on Mammographic Breast Parenchymal Density," *Journal of Clinical Oncology* 15 (1997): 3201–7.

23   E. Lundström et al., "Mammographic Breast Density during Hormone Replacement Therapy: Effects of Continuous Combination, Unopposed Transdermal and Low-Potency Estrogen Regimens," *Climacteric* 4, no. 1 (March 2001): 42–48.

24   Carney et al., "Individual and Combined Effects," 168–75.

25   J. A. Harvey, "The Mammogram in Menopause: How Hormones Influence Imaging," *Menopausal Medicine* 8 (Spring 2000): 5–9

26   M. B. Laya et al., "Effect of Estrogen Replacement Therapy on the Specificity and Sensitivity of Screening Mammography," *Journal of the National Cancer Institute* 88 (1996): 643–49.

27   "BRCA1 and BRCA2: Cancer Risk and Genetic Testing," National Cancer Institute, last modified April 1, 2015, cancer.gov/about-cancer/causes -prevention/genetics/brca-fact-sheet.

28   American Cancer Society, "Breast Cancer Facts & Figures, 2013–2014," accessed September 25, 2015, cancer.org/acs/groups/content/@research/documents /document/acspc-042725.pdf.

29   S. Chen and G. Parmigiani, "Meta-Analysis of BRCA1 and BRCA2 Penetrance," *Journal of Clinical Oncology* 25, no. 11 (2007): 1329–33.

30   A. Jolie Pitt, "Angelina Jolie Pitt: Diary of a Surgery," *New York Times* (March 24, 2015), A23.

31 L. T. Shuster et al., "Prophylactic Oophorectomy in Premenopausal Women and Long-Term Health," *Menopause International* 14, no. 3 (September 2008): 111–16.

32 pancan.org/reports/report-the-alarming-rise-of-pancreatic-cancer-deaths-in -the-u-s-2/.

33 W. A. Roca et al., "Increased Risk of Cognitive Impairment or Dementia in Women Who Underwent Oophorectomy before Menopause," *Neurology* 69, no. 11 (September 11, 2007): 1074–83.

34 E. Løkkegaard et al., "The Association between Early Menopause and Risk of Ischaemic Heart Disease: Influence of Hormone Therapy," *Maturitas* 53, no. 2 (January 20, 2006): 226–33.

35 C. M. Rivera et al., "Increased Cardiovascular Mortality after Early Bilateral Oophorectomy," *Menopause* 16, no. 1 (January–February 2009): 15–23.

36 G. L. Anderson, M. Limacher, A. R. Assaf et al., "Effects of Conjugated Equine Estrogen in Postmenopausal Women with Hysterectomy: The Women's Health Initiative Randomized Controlled Trial," *JAMA* 291, no. 14 (April 14, 2004): 1701–12.

37 R. S. Cecchin et al., "Body Mass Index and the Risk for Developing Invasive Breast Cancer among High-Risk Women in NSABP P-1 and STAR Breast Cancer Prevention Trials," *Cancer Prevention Research* 5, no. 4 (April 2012): 583–92.

38 W. Somboonporn, S. Panna, T. Temtanakitpaisan, et al., "Effects of the Levonorgestrel-Releasing Intrauterine System Plus Estrogen Therapy in Perimenopausal and Postmenopausal Women: Systematic Review and Meta-Analysis," *Menopause* 18, no. 10 (October 2011): 1060–66.

39 M. M. Gaudet et al., "Active Smoking and Breast Cancer Risk: Original Cohort Data and Meta-Analysis," *Journal of the National Cancer Institute* 105, no. 8 (April 17, 2013): 515–25.

40 C. M. Friedenreich et al., "Effects of a High vs Moderate Volume of Aerobic Exercise on Adiposity Outcomes in Postmenopausal Women: A Randomized Clinical Trial," *JAMA Oncology* 1, no. 6 (September 2015): 766–76.

41 "Exercise," Breastcancer.org, last modified January 30, 2015, breastcancer.org /tips/exercise.

42 "Breast Cancer Prevention and Early Detection," American Cancer Society, last modified October 20, 2015, cancer.org/cancer/breastcancer/moreinformation /breastcancerearlydetection/index.

Chapter 5: The Estrogen Fix and Your Heart

1 "Cardiovascular Diseases (CVDs)," World Health Organization, last modified January 2015, who.int/mediacentre/factsheets/fs317/en.

2 A. L. Hersh, M. L. Stefanick, and R. S. Stafford, "National Use of Postmenopausal Hormone Therapy: Annual Trends and Response to Recent Evidence," *JAMA* 291, no. 1 (2004): 47–53.

3 R. K. Dubey et al., "Vascular Consequences of Menopause and Hormone Therapy: Importance of Timing of Treatment and Type of Estrogen," *Cardiovascular Research* 66, no. 2 (May 1, 2005): 295–300.

4   "ACOG Recommends Vaginal Hysterectomy as Approach of Choice," American College of Obstetricians and Gynecologists, October 21, 2009, acog. org/About-ACOG/News-Room/News-Releases/2009/ACOG-Recommends -Vaginal-Hysterectomy-as-Approach-of-Choice.

5   H. Keshavarz et al., "Hysterectomy Surveillance–United States, 1994–1999," *Morbidity and Mortality Weekly Report* 51 (July 12, 2002): 1–8, cdc.gov/mmwr /preview/mmwrhtml/ss5105a1.htm.

6   T. C. Okeke, U. B. Anyaehie, and C. C. Ezenyeaku, "Premature Menopause," *Annals of Medical & Health Sciences Research* 3, no. 1 (January–March 2013): 90–95.

7   J. E. Rossouw, G. L. Anderson, R. L. Prentice et al., "Risks and Benefits of Estrogen Plus Progestin in Healthy Postmenopausal Women: Principal Results from the Women's Health Initiative," *JAMA* 288, no. 3 (July 17, 2002): 321–33.

8   L. Rapaport, "Wyeth, J&J Drugs Cut Menopause Symptoms in Studies (Update2)," *Bloomberg.com*, May 8, 2007, bloomberg.com/apps/news?pid =newsarchive&sid=aY_IrK7En164.

9   P. M. Sarrel et al., "The Mortality Toll of Estrogen Avoidance: An Analysis of Excess Deaths among Hysterectomized Women Aged 5059 Years," *American Journal of Public Health* 103, no. 9 (September 2013): 1583–88.

10 G. L. Anderson et al., "Effects of Conjugated Equine Estrogen in Postmenopausal Women with Hysterectomy: The Women's Health Initiative Randomized Controlled Trial," *JAMA* 291, no. 14 (April 14, 2004): 1701–12.

11 A. Z. LaCroix et al., "Health Outcomes after Stopping Conjugated Equine Estrogens among Postmenopausal Women with Prior Hysterectomy: A Randomized Controlled Trial," *JAMA* 305, no. 13 (April 6, 2011): 1305–14.

12 T. S. Mikkola, P. Tuomikoski, H. Lyytinen et al., "Estradiol-Based Postmenopausal Hormone Therapy and Risk of Cardiovascular and All-Cause Mortality," *Menopause* 22, no. 9 (September 2015): 976–83.

13 T. S. Mikkola, P. Tuomikoski, H. Lyytinen, et al., "Increased Cardiovascular Mortality Risk in Women Discontinuing Postmenopausal Hormone Therapy," *The Journal of Clinical Endocrinology & Metabolism* 100, no. 12 (December 2015): 4588–94.

14 A. M. Kaunitz and J. E. Manson, "Failure to Treat Menopausal Symptoms: A Disconnect Between Clinical Practice and Scientific Data," *Menopause* 22, no. 7 (July 2015): 687–88.

15 D. J. DeNoon, "The 10 Most Prescribed Drugs: Most-Prescribed Drug List Differs from List of Drugs with Biggest Market Share," WebMD, April 20, 2011, webmd.com/news/20110420/the-10-most-prescribed-drugs.

16 "Guidelines Resource Center," American Heart Association, last modified September 4, 2015, heart.org/HEARTORG/Conditions/Understanding-the -New-Prevention Guidelines_UCM_458155_Article.jsp.

17 A. Wakatsuki et al., "Estrogen-Induced Small Low Density Lipoprotein Particles May Be Atherogenic in Postmenopausal Women," *Journal of the American College of Cardiology* 37, no. 2 (February 2001): 425–30.

18 "Cardiovascular Diseases (CVDs)," World Health Organization, last modified January 2015, who.int/mediacentre/factsheets/fs317/en.

19   A. Wakatsuki, N. Ikenoue, and Y. Sagara, "Estrogen-Induced Small Low-Density Lipoprotein Particles in Postmenopausal Women," *Obstetrics & Gynecology* 91, no. 2 (February 1998): 234–40.

20   A. Wakatsuki et al., "Different Effects of Oral Conjugated Equine Estrogen and Transdermal Estrogen Replacement Therapy on Size and Oxidative Susceptibility of Low-Density Lipoprotein Particles in Postmenopausal Women," *Circulation* 106, no. 14 (October 1, 2002): 1771–76.

21   A. Paganini-Hill, R. Dworsky, and R. M. Krauss, "Hormone Replacement Therapy, Hormone Levels, and Lipoprotein Cholesterol Concentrations in Elderly Women," *American Journal of Obstetrics and Gynecology* 174, no. 3 (March 1996): 897–902.

22   A. Sierra-Ramirez et al., "Acute Effects of Testosterone on Intracellular Ca2+ Kinetics in Rat Coronary Endothelial Cells Are Exerted via Aromatization to Estrogens," *American Journal of Physiology—Heart and Circulatory Physiology* 287, no. 1 (2004): H63–71.

23   A. Gougelet et al., "Oestrogen Receptors Pathways to Oestrogen Responsive Elements: The Transactivation Function-1 Acts as the Keystone of Oestrogen Receptor (ER) Beta-Mediated Transcriptional Repression of ERalpha," *Journal of Steroid Biochemistry and Molecular Biology* 104, no. 3–5 (May 2007): 110–22.

24   K. Kublickiene et al., "Small Artery Endothelial Dysfunction in Postmenopausal Women: In Vitro Function, Morphology, and Modification by Estrogen and Selective Estrogen Receptor Modulators," *Journal of Clinical Endocrinology & Metabolism* 90, no. 11 (November 2005): 6113–22.

25   C. Vitale et al., "Time Since Menopause Influences the Acute and Chronic Effect of Estrogens on Endothelial Function," *Arteriosclerosis, Thrombosis, and Vascular Biology* 28, no. 2 (February 2008): 348–52.

26   V. Guetta and R. O. Cannon III, "Cardiovascular Effects of Estrogen and Lipid Lowering Therapies in Postmenopausal Women," *Circulation* 93 (1996): 1928–37.

27   R. A. Lobo, "Effects of Hormonal Replacement on Lipids and Lipoproteins in Postmenopausal Women," *Journal of Clinical Endocrinology & Metabolism* 73, no. 5 (1991): 925–930.

28   B. W. Walsh et al., "Effects of Postmenopausal Estrogen Replacement on the Concentrations and Metabolism of Plasma Lipoproteins," *New England Journal of Medicine* 325 (1991): 1196–1204.

29   P. Collins et al., "17β-Estradiol Attenuates Acetylcholine-Induced Coronary Arterial Constriction in Women but Not Men with Coronary Heart Disease," *Circulation* 92 (1995): 24–30.

30   D. M. Gilligan, A. A. Quyyumi, and R. O. Cannon, "Effects of Physiological Levels of Estrogen on Coronary Vasomotor Function in Postmenopausal Women," *Circulation* 89 (1994): 2545–51.

31   "Menopause and Heart Disease," American Heart Association, last modified July 2015, heart.org/HEARTORG/Conditions/More/MyHeartandStroke News /Menopause-and-Heart-Disease_UCM_448432_Article.jsp.

32   "Early Menopause Associated with Increased Risk of Heart Disease, Stroke,"
     Johns Hopkins Medicine, September 18, 2012, hopkinsmedicine.org/news
     /media/releases/early_menopause_associated_with_increased_risk_of_heart
     _disease_stroke.

33   O. M. Reslan and R. A. Khalil, "Vascular Effects of Estrogenic Menopausal
     Hormone Therapy," *Reviews on Recent Clinical Trials* 7, no. 1 (February 1, 2012):
     47–70.

34   W. B. Kannel et al., "Menopause and Risk of Cardiovascular Disease: The
     Framingham Study," *Annals of Internal Medicine* 85 (1976): 447–52.

35   L. Rosenberg et al., "Early Menopause and the Risk of Myocardial Infarction,"
     American Journal of Obstetrics and Gynecology 139, no. 1 (January 1981): 47–51.

36   G. A. Colditz et al., "Menopause and the Risk of Coronary Heart Disease in
     Women," *New England Journal of Medicine* 316, no. 18 (April 30, 1987): 1105–10.

37   W. J. Mack et al., "Elevated Subclinical Atherosclerosis Associated with
     Oophorectomy Is Related to Time Since Menopause Rather Than Type of
     Menopause," *Fertility and Sterility* 82, no. 2 (August 2004): 391–97.

38   R. K. Dubey et al., "Vascular Consequences of Menopause and Hormone
     Therapy: Importance of Timing of Treatment and Type of Estrogen,"
     Cardiovascular Research 66, no. 2 (May 1, 2005): 295–306.

39   Reslan and Khalil, "Estrogenic Menopausal Hormone Therapy," 47–70.

40   K. Sutton-Tyrrell et al., "Carotid Atherosclerosis in Premenopausal and
     Postmenopausal Women and Its Association with Risk Factors Measured after
     Menopause," *Stroke* 29, no. 6 (June 1998): 1116–21.

41   H. W. Peters et al., "Menopausal Status and Risk Factors for Cardiovascular
     Disease," *Journal of Internal Medicine* 246, no. 6 (December 1999): 521–28.

42   Mack et al., "Elevated Subclinical Atherosclerosis," 391–97.

43   M. E. Mendelsohn and R. H. Karas, "Molecular and Cellular Basis of
     Cardiovascular Gender Differences," *Science* 308, no. 5728 (June 10, 2005):
     1583–87.

44   T. S. Mikkola, P. Tuomikoski, H. Lyytinen, et al., "Estradiol-Based
     Postmenopausal Hormone Therapy and Risk of Cardiovascular and All-Cause
     Mortality," *Menopause* 22, no. 9 (September 2015): 976–83.

45   F. Grodstein et al., "A Prospective, Observational Study of Postmenopausal
     Hormone Therapy and Primary Prevention of Cardiovascular Disease," *Annals
     of Internal Medicine* 133, no. 12 (December 19, 2000): 933–41.

46   Ibid.

47   F. Grodstein, J. E. Manson, and M. J. Stampfer, "Hormone Therapy and
     Coronary Heart Disease: The Role of Time Since Menopause and Age at
     Hormone Initiation," *Journal of Women's Health & Gender-Based Medicine* 15, no.
     1 (January–February 2006): 35–44.

48   T. S. Mikkola and T. B. Clarkson, "Estrogen Replacement Therapy,
     Atherosclerosis, and Vascular Function," *Cardiovascular Research* 53, no. 3
     (February 15, 2002): 605–19.

49 J. K. Williams et al., "Regression of Atherosclerosis in Female Monkeys," *Arteriosclerosis, Thrombosis, and Vascular Biology* 15, no. 7 (July 1995): 827–36.

50 T. Mori et al., "Effects of Short-Term Estrogen Treatment on the Neointimal Response to Balloon Injury of Rat Carotid Artery," *American Journal of Cardiology* 85, no. 10 (May 15, 2000): 1276–79.

51 G. L. Anderson et al., "Effects of Conjugated Equine Estrogen in Postmenopausal Women with Hysterectomy: The Women's Health Initiative Randomized Controlled Trial," *JAMA* 291, no. 14 (April 14, 2004): 1701–12.

52 A. Z. LaCroix et al., "Health Outcomes after Stopping Conjugated Equine Estrogens among Postmenopausal Women with Prior Hysterectomy: A Randomized Controlled Trial," *JAMA* 305, no. 13 (April 6, 2011): 1305–14.

53 D. O. Stram et al., "Age-Specific Effects of Hormone Therapy Use on Overall Mortality and Ischemic Heart Disease Mortality among Women in the California Teachers Study," *Menopause* 18, no. 3 (March 2011): 253–61.

54 M. Wellons et al., "Early Menopause Predicts Future Coronary Heart Disease and Stroke: The Multi-Ethnic Study of Atherosclerosis (MESA)," *Menopause* 19, no. 10 (October 2012): 1081–87.

55 P. M. Sarrel et al., "The Mortality Toll of Estrogen Avoidance: An Analysis of Excess Deaths among Hysterectomized Women Aged 50 to 59 Years," *American Journal of Public Health* 103, no. 9 (September 2013): 1583–88.

Chapter 6: The Estrogen Fix and Your Brain

1 T. Lewis, "How Men's Brains Are Wired Differently Than Women's," *Scientific American*, December 2, 2013, scientificamerican.com/article/how-mens-brains-are-wired-differently-than-women.

2 B. S. McKuen and B. S. Alves, "Estrogen Actions in the Central Nervous System," *Endocrine Reviews* 20, no. 3 (June 1999): 279–307.

3 Ibid.

4 J. S. M. Archer, "Estrogen and Mood Change via CNS Activity," *Menopausal Medicine* 7, no. 3 (Fall 1999): 4–8.

5 American Physiological Society, "Moderate Exercise Improves Brain Blood Flow in Elderly Women," www.the-aps.org/mm/hp/Audiences/Public-Press/Archive/2011/9.html.

6 M. Penotti et al., "Cerebral Artery Blood Flow in Relation to Age and Menopausal Status," *Obstetrics & Gynecology* 88 (July 1996): 106–9.

7 B. Cacciatore et al., "Randomized Comparison of Oral and Transdermal Hormone Replacement on Carotid and Uterine Artery Resistance to Blood Flow," *Obstetrics & Gynecology* 92 (October 1998): 563–68.

8 C. Zhang, "The Role of Inflammatory Cytokines in Endothelial Dysfunction," *Basic Research in Cardiology* 103, no. 5 (September 2008): 398–406.

9 D. A. Smiley and R. A. Khalil, "Estrogenic Compounds, Estrogen Receptors and Vascular Cell Signaling in the Aging Blood Vessels," *Current Medicinal Chemistry* 16, no. 15 (2009): 1863–87.

10   A. Wnuk, D. L. Korol, and K. I. Erickson, "Estrogens, Hormone Therapy, and Hippocampal Volume in Postmenopausal Women," *Maturitas* 73, no. 3 (November 2012): 186–190.

11   G. P. Dohanich, D. L. Korol, and T. J. Shors, "Steroids and Cognition," in *Hormones, Brain and Behavior*, 2nd ed., ed. D. Pfaff et al. (New York, NY: Academic Press, 2009), 539–76.

12   R. Schmidt et al., "Estrogen Replacement Therapy in Older Women: A Neuropsychological and Brain MRI Study," *Journal of the American Geriatric Society* 44, no. 11 (November 1996): 1307–13.

13   B. B. Sherwin, "Estrogen and/or Androgen Replacement Therapy and Cognitive Functioning in Surgically Menopausal Women," *Psychoneuroendocrinology* 13, no. 4 (1988): 345–57.

14   T. Duka, R. Tasker, and J. F. McGowan, "The Effects of 3-Week Estrogen Hormone Replacement on Cognition in Elderly Healthy Females," *Psychopharmacology* 149, no. 2 (2000): 129–39.

15   M. Boccardi et al., "Effects of Hormone Therapy on Brain Morphology of Healthy Postmenopausal Women: A Voxel-Based Morphometry Study," *Menopause* 13, no. 4 (July–August 2006): 584–91.

16   "Mayo Clinic Research Shows Estrogen Protects Women's Brains Prior to Menopause; Ovary Removal before Menopause Increases Risk of Parkinson's Disease and Parkinsonism," Drugs.com, August 29, 2007, drugs.com/clinical _trials/mayo-clinic-research-shows-estrogen-protects-women-s-brains-prior -menopause-ovary-removal-before-1816.html.

17   S. M. Phillips and B. B. Sheridan, "Effects of Estrogen on Memory Function in Surgically Menopausal Women," *Psychoneuroendocrinology* 17, no. 5 (1992): 485–95.

18   L. J. Currie et al., "Postmenopausal Estrogen Use Affects Risk for Parkinson Disease," *Archives of Neurology* 61, no. 6 (June 2004): 886–88.

19   C. Iadecola and M. Alexander, "Cerebral Ischemia and Inflammation," *Current Opinion in Neurology* 14, no. 1 (February 2001): 89–94.

20   J. R. Meendering et al., "Estrogen, Medroxyprogesterone Acetate, Endothelial Function, and Biomarkers of Cardiovascular Risk in Young Women," *American Journal of Physiology–Heart and Circulatory Physiology* 294, no. 4 (April 2008): H1630–37.

21   "Depo-Provera Birth Control Might Raise Breast Cancer Risk," *U.S. News & World Report*, April 4, 2012, health.usnews.com/health-news/news/articles /2012/04/04/depo-provera-birth-control-might-raise-breast-cancer-risk.

22   F. Kronenberg, "Hot Flashes: Epidemiology and Physiology," *Annals of the New York Academy of Sciences* 592 (1990): 123–133.

23   R. A. Greene et al., "Comparison between Regional Cerebral Blood Flow in Hypoestrogenic Women and Patients with Alzheimer's Disease–A Descriptive Study," *Neurobiology of Aging* 10, no. 4 (1998): S180.

24   Ibid.

25   R. Peters, "Ageing and the Brain," *Postgraduate Medical Journal* 82, no. 964 (February 2006): 84–88.

26   R. I. Scahill et al., "A Longitudinal Study of Brain Volume Changes in Normal Aging Using Serial Registered Magnetic Resonance Imaging," *Archives of Neurology* 60, no. 7 (July 2003): 989–94.

27   J. Compton, T. van Amelsvoort, and D. Murphy, "HRT and Its Effect on Normal Ageing of the Brain and Dementia," *British Journal of Clinical Pharmacology* 52, no. 6 (December 2001): 647–53.

28   D. G. Murphy et al., "Sex Differences in Human Brain Morphometry and Metabolism: An In Vivo Quantitative Magnetic Resonance Imaging and Positron Emission Tomography Study on the Effect of Aging," *Archives of General Psychiatry* 53, no. 7 (July 1996): 585–94.

29   Compton, van Amelsvoort, and Murphy, "HRT and Its Effect," 647–53.

30   Murphy et al., "Sex Differences in Human Brain Morphometry," 585–94.

31   R. L. Ferrini and E. L. Barrett-Connor, "Sex Hormones and Age: A Cross-Sectional Study of Testosterone and Estradiol and Their Bioavailable Fractions in Community-Dwelling Men," *American Journal of Epidemiology* 147, no. 8 (1998): 750–54.

32   T. E. Wroolie et al., "Differences in Verbal Memory Performance in Postmenopausal Women Receiving Hormone Therapy: 17β-Estradiol versus Conjugated Equine Estrogens," *American Journal of Geriatric Psychiatry* 19, no. 9 (September 2011): 792–802.

33   S. E. Shaywitz et al., "Effect of Estrogen on Brain Activation Patterns in Postmenopausal Women during Working Memory Tasks," *JAMA* 281, no. 13 (1999): 1197–202.

34   H. Joffe et al., "Estrogen Therapy Selectively Enhances Prefrontal Cognitive Processes: A Randomized, Double-Blind, Placebo-Controlled Study with Functional Magnetic Resonance Imaging in Perimenopausal and Recently Postmenopausal Women," *Menopause* 13, no. 3 (2006): 411–22.

35   E. Vegeto, P. Ciana, and A. Maggi, "Estrogen and Inflammation: Hormone Generous Action Spreads to the Brain," *Molecular Psychiatry* 7, no. 3 (2002): 236–38.

36   U. Halbreich et al., "Possible Acceleration of Age Effects on Cognition Following Menopause," *Journal of Psychiatric Research* 29, no. 3 (1995): 153–63.

37   M. Di Bari, J. Williamson, and M. Pahor, "Missing Data in Epidemiological Studies of Age-Associated Cognitive Decline," *Journal of the American Geriatrics Society* 47, no. 11 (1999): 1380–81.

38   R. Honkanen, M. Komulainon, and K. Honkanen, "Hormone Replacement Therapy Prevents Falls in Early Postmenopausal Women," abstract, European Congress on Osteoporosis 286 (1998).

39   Centers for Disease Control and Prevention, National Center for Injury Prevention and Control. Web-based Injury Statistics Query and Reporting System (WISQARS) [online]. Accessed August 15, 2013. www.cdc.gov /injury/wisqars/index.html.

40   "Menopause and Mental Health," Womenshealth.gov, last modified September 29, 2010, womenshealth.gov/menopause/menopause-mental-health.

41   L. T. Shuster et al., "Premature Menopause or Early Menopause: Long-Term Health Consequences," *Maturitas* 65, no. 2 (February 2010): 161.

42   J. D. Wright, T. J. Herzog, J. Tsui, et al., "Nationwide Trends in the Performance of Hysterectomy in the United States," *Obstetrics & Gynecology* 122, no. 2 Pt. 1 (August 2013): 233–41.

43   H. Keshavarz et al., "Hysterectomy Surveillance–United States, 1994–1999," *Morbidity and Mortality Weekly Report* 51 (July 12, 2002): 1–8, cdc.gov/mmwr /preview/mmwrhtml/ss5105a1.htm.

44   S. L. Davison et al., "Androgen Levels in Adult Females: Changes with Age, Menopause, and Oophorectomy," *Journal of Clinical Endocrinology & Metabolism* 90, no. 7 (2005): 3847–53.

45   M. Conrad Stoppler, "Menopause Q&A by Dr. Stoppler," MedicineNet.com, last modified June 6, 2014, medicinenet.com/script/main/art.asp?articlekey =77937.

46   C. M. Farquhar et al., "The Association of Hysterectomy and Menopause: A Prospective Cohort Study," *BJOG: An International Journal of Obstetrics and Gynaecology* 112, no. 7 (July 2005): 956–62.

47   P. M. Sarrel, S. D. Sullivan, L. M. Nelson, "Hormone Replacement Therapy in Young Women with Surgical Primary Ovarian Insufficiency," *Fertility and Sterility* 106, no. 7 (December 2016): 1580–87.

48   G. L. Gierach et al., "Long-Term Overall and Disease-Specific Mortality Associated with Benign Gynecologic Surgery Performed at Different Ages," *Menopause* 21, no. 6 (June 2014): 592–601.

49   O. Harmanli et al., "Obstetrician-Gynecologists' Opinions on Elective Bilateral Oophorectomy at the Time of Hysterectomy in the United States: A Nationwide Survey," *Menopause* 21, no. 4 (April 2014): 355–60.

50   P. P. Zandi et al., "Hormone Replacement Therapy and Incidence of Alzheimer Disease in Older Women: The Cache County Study," *JAMA* 288, no. 17 (2002): 2123–29.

51   W. Xu et al., "Meta-Analysis of Modifiable Risk Factors for Alzheimer's Disease," *Journal of Neurology, Neurosurgery & Psychiatry*, published electronically August 20, 2015.

52   L. S. Cohen et al., "Risk for New Onset of Depression during the Menopausal Transition: The Harvard Study of Moods and Cycles," *Archives of General Psychiatry* 63, no. 4 (2006): 385–90.

53   D. Goleman, "The Brain Manages Happiness and Sadness in Different Centers," *New York Times*, March 28, 1995, nytimes.com/1995/03/28/science /the-brain-manages-happiness-and-sadness-in-different-centers.html.

54 www.nlm.nih.gov/medlineplus/news/fullstory_153295.html.

55 B. L. Harlow et al., "Depression and Its Influence on Reproductive Endocrine and Menstrual Cycle Markers Associated with Perimenopause: The Harvard Study of Moods and Cycles," *Archives of General Psychiatry* 60, no. 1 (2003): 29–36.

56 C. N. Soares et al., "Efficacy of Estradiol for the Treatment of Depressive Disorders in Perimenopausal Women: A Double-Blind, Randomized, Placebo-Controlled Trial," *Archives of General Psychiatry* 58, no. 6 (June 2001): 529–34.

57 C. N. Soares et al., "Efficacy of Citalopram as a Monotherapy or as an Adjunctive Treatment to Estrogen Therapy for Perimenopausal and Postmenopausal Women with Depression and Vasomotor Symptoms," *Journal of Clinical Psychiatry* 64, no. 4 (April 2003): 473–79.

58 M. D. Gershon and J. Tack, "The Serotonin Signaling System: From Basic Understanding to Drug Development for Functional GI Disorders," *Gastroenterology* 132, no. 1 (2007): 397–414.

59 J. C. Bornstein, "Serotonin in the Gut: What Does It Do?" *Frontiers in Neuroscience,* published electronically February 6, 2012.

60 "A Healthy Gut Balances Moods?" Body Ecology, Inc., accessed October 23, 2015, bodyecology.com/articles/a-healthy-gut-balances-moods.

61 C. B. Zhu et al., "Interleukin-1 Receptor Activation by Systemic Lipopolysaccharide Induces Behavioral Despair Linked to MAPK Regulation of CNS Serotonin Transporters," *Neuropsychopharmacology* 35, no. 13 (2010): 2510–20.

62 G. P. Ahern, "5-HT and the Immune System," *Current Opinion in Pharmacology* 11, no. 1 (February 2011): 29–33.

63 Zhu et al., "Interleukin-1 Receptor Activation," 2510–20.

64 B. J. Fuhrman et al., "Associations of the Fecal Microbiome with Urinary Estrogens and Estrogen Metabolites in Postmenopausal Women," *Journal of Clinical Endocrinology & Metabolism* 99, no. 12 (December 2014): 2222.

65 Fuhrman et al., 4632–40.

66 "Depression," Vitamin D Council, last modified June 2013, vitamindcouncil.org /health-conditions/depression.

67 D. K. Hall-Flavin, "What's the Relationship between Vitamin B-12 and Depression?" Mayo Clinic, February 6, 2014, mayoclinic.org/diseases-conditions /depression/expert-answers/vitamin-b12-and-depression/FAQ-20058077.

68 medscape.com/viewarticle/406718_2.

69 Xu et al., "Meta-Analysis of Modifiable Risk Factors," doi:10.1136/jnnp-2015 -310548.

70 K. Yaffe et al., "Association between Bone Mineral Density and Cognitive Decline in Older Women," *Journal of the American Geriatrics Society* 47, no. 10 (1999): 1176–82.

71 W. A. Rocca et al., "Increased Risk of Cognitive Impairment or Dementia in Women Who Underwent Oophorectomy before Menopause," *Neurology* 69, no. 11 (September 11, 2007): 1074–83.

72 E. G. Jacobs et al., "Accelerated Cell Aging in Female APOE-ε4 Carriers: Implications for Hormone Therapy Use," *PLOS ONE* 8, no. 2 (February 13, 2013): e54713.

73 Y. Xu, T. P. Nedungadi, L. Zhu, et al., "Distinct Hypothalamic Neurons Mediate Estrogenic Effects on Energy Homeostasis and Reproduction," *Cell Metabolism* 14, no. 4 (October 2011): 453–65.

74 H. Attarian et al., "Treatment of Chronic Insomnia Disorder in Menopause: Evaluation of Literature," *Menopause* 22, no. 6 (2015): 674–84.

75 A. M. De Fonsecca et al., "Impact of Age and Body Mass on the Intensity of Menopausal Symptoms in 5968 Brazilian Women," *Gynecological Endocrinology* 29, no. 2 (2013): 116–18.

76 E. Vousoura et al., "Vasomotor and Depression Symptoms May Be Associated with Different Sleep Disturbance Patterns in Postmenopausal Women," *Menopause* 22, no. 10 (October 2015): 1053–57.

77 S. Taheri et al., "Short Sleep Duration Is Associated with Reduced Leptin, Elevated Ghrelin, and Increased Body Mass Index," *PLOS Medicine* 1, no. 3 (December 7, 2004): e62.

78 United States Congress Joint Economic Committee, *Women and the Economy 2010: 25 Years of Progress but Challenges Remain*, August 2010, jec.senate.gov /public/_cache/files/f9f3a9b8-2f54-4e83-9029-477a3fc73cd5/women-and-the -economy-2010---25-years-of-progress-but-challenges-remain.pdf.

79 "Women in the Labor Force," US Department of Labor, accessed October 23, 2015, dol.gov/wb/stats/stats_data.htm.

80 J. Ilmairinen, *Towards a Longer Worklife! Ageing and the Quality of Worklife in the European Union* (Helsinki, Finland: Helsinki and Finnish Institute of Occupation Health, Ministry of Social Affairs and Health, 2005).

81 P. M. Sarrel, "Women, Work, and Menopause," *Menopause* 19, no. 3 (March 2012): 250–52.

82 T. A. Barmby, M. G. Ercolani, and J. G. Treble, "Sickness Absence: An International Comparison," *Economic Journal* 112, no. 480 (June 2002): F315–31.

83 G. Wynne-Jones et al., "Identification of UK Sickness Certification Rates, Standardized for Age and Sex," *British Journal of General Practice* 59, no. 564 (2009): 510–16.

84 M. Geukes et al., "The Impact of Menopausal Symptoms on Work Ability," *Menopause* 19, no. 3 (2012): 278–82.

85 B. Ayers and M. S. Hunter, "Health-Related Quality of Life of Women with Menopausal Hot Flushes and Night Sweats," *Climacteric* 16, no. 2 (April 2013): 235–9.

86 A. Oldenhave et al., "Impact of Climacteric on Well-Being: A Survey Based on 5213 Women 39 to 60 Years Old," *American Journal of Obstetrics and Gynecology* 168, no. 3 (1993): 772–80.

87 P. Sarrel et al., "Ovarian Steroids and the Capacity to Function at Home and in the Workplace," *Annals of the New York Academy of Sciences* 592 (June 1990): 156–61.

88   J. A. Simon and K. Z. Reape, "Understanding the Menopausal Experiences of Professional Women," *Menopause* 16, no. 1 (2009): 73–76.

89   Sarrel, "Women, Work, and Menopause," 250–52.

90   S. A. Tsai, M. L. Stefanick, and R. S. Stafford. "Trends in Menopausal Hormone Use of US Office-Based Physicians, 2000–2009," *Menopause* 18, no. 4 (2011): 385–92.

91   D. Searcey, "For Women in Midlife, Career Gains Slip Away," *New York Times*, June 23, 2014, nytimes.com/2014/06/24/business/women-leave-their-careers-in -peak-years.html.

92   P. Sarrel et al., "Incremental Direct and Indirect Costs of Untreated Vasomotor," *Menopause* 22, no. 3 (March 2015): 260–66.

93   G. S. Passos et al., "Exercise Improves Immune Function, Antidepressive Response, and Sleep Quality in Patients with Chronic Primary Insomnia," *BioMed Research International* 2014 (September 21, 2014). www.hindawi.com /journals/bmri/2014/498961/citations.

94   G. S. Passos et al., "Effect of Acute Physical Exercise on Patients with Chronic Primary Insomnia," *Journal of Clinical Sleep Medicine* 6, no. 3 (2010): 270–75.

95   G. S. Passos et al., "Effects of Moderate Aerobic Exercise Training on Chronic Primary Insomnia," *Sleep Medicine* 12, no. 10 (2011): 1018–27.

96   K. J. Reid et al., "Aerobic Exercise Improves Self-Reported Sleep and Quality of Life in Older Adults with Insomnia," *Sleep Medicine* 11, no. 9 (2010): 934–40.

Chapter 7: The Estrogen Fix and Your Bones

1   Y. Imai et al., "Estrogens Maintain Bone Mass by Regulating Expression of Genes Controlling Function and Life Span in Mature Osteoclasts," *Annals of the New York Academy of Sciences* 1173, supplement 1 (September 2009): E31–39.

2   E. M. Haas, "Minerals: Calcium," Healthy.net, accessed October 23, 2015, healthy.net/scr/Article.aspx?Id=2019.

3   parathyroid.com/parathyroid-function.htm.

4   E. Damien, J. S. Price, and L. E. Lanyon, "Mechanical Strain Stimulates Osteoblast Proliferation through the Estrogen Receptor in Males as well as Females," *Journal of Bone and Mineral Research* 15, no. 11 (November 2000): 2169–77.

5   R. Lindsay, "The Menopause: Sex Steroids and Osteoporosis," *Clinical Obstetrics and Gynecology* 30, no. 4 (1987): 847–59.

6   B. L. Riggs, "The Mechanisms of Estrogen Regulation of Bone Resorption," *Journal of Clinical Investigation* 106, no. 10 (2000): 1203–4.

7   S. C. Manolagas, "Birth and Death of Bone Cells: Basic Regulatory Mechanisms and Implications for the Pathogenesis and Treatment of Osteoporosis," *Endocrine Reviews* 21, no. 2 (2000): 115–37.

8   Riggs, "The Mechanisms of Estrogen Regulation," 1203–4.

9   R. Pacifici, "Cytokines, and Pathogenesis of Postmenopausal Osteoporosis," *Journal of Bone and Mineral Research* 11, no. 8 (1996): 1043–51.

10   T. Nakamura, "Estrogen Prevents Bone Loss via Estrogen Receptor Alpha and Induction of Fas Ligand in Osteoclasts," *Cell* 130, no. 5 (September 7, 2007): 811–23.

11   R. Lindsay and F. Cosman, "Estrogen," in *The Aging Skeleton*, ed. C. J. Rosen, J. Glowacki, and J. P. Bilezikian (Waltham, MA: Academic Press, 1999), 495–505.

12   E. Rosenthal, "Hormone Therapy Seen to Cut Risk of Broken Hip," *New York Times*, July 16, 1990, nytimes.com/1990/07/16/us/hormone-therapy-seen-to-cut -risk-of-broken-hip.html.

13   "Bone Health," University of Texas MD Anderson Cancer Center, accessed October 24, 2015, mdanderson.org/patient-and-cancer-information/cancer -information/cancer-topics/dealing-with-cancer-treatment/bone-health /index.html.

14   S. D. Sullivan et al., "Effects of Self-Reported Age of Non-Surgical Menopause on Time to First Fracture and Bone Mineral Density in the Women's Health Initiative Observational Study," *Menopause* 22, no. 10 (October 2015): 1035–44.

15   mayoclinic.org/diseases-conditions/high-blood-pressure/in-depth/calcium -channel-blockers/art-20047605.

16   "Calcium Supplements: Who Should Take Calcium Supplements?" MedlinePlus, last modified October 21, 2015, https://www.nlm.nih.gov /medlineplus/ency/article/007477.htm.

17   Haas, "Minerals: Calcium," healthy.net/scr/Article.aspx?Id=2019.

18   S. Gandini et al., "Meta-Analysis of Observational Studies of Serum 25-Hydroxyvitamin D Levels and Colorectal, Breast and Prostate Cancer and Colorectal Adenoma," *International Journal of Cancer* 128, no. 6 (2011): 1414–24.

19   "Vitamin D and Cancer Prevention," National Cancer Institute, last modified October 21, 2013, cancer.gov/about-cancer/causes-prevention/risk/diet /vitamin-d-fact-sheet.

20   A. R. Martineau, D. A. Jolliffe, R. L. Hooper, et al., "Vitamin D supplementation to Prevent Acute Respiratory Tract Infections: Systematic Review And Meta-Analysis of Individual Participant Data," *BMJ* 356 (February 15, 2017): i6583; M. Urashima, T. Segawa, M. Segawa, et al., "Randomized Trial of Vitamin D Supplementation to Prevent Seasonal Influenza A in Schoolchildren," *American Journal of Clinical Nutrition* 91, no. 5 (May 2010): 1255–60.

21   D. Agnusdei et al., "Calcitonin and Estrogens," *Journal of Endocrinological Investigation* 13, no. 8 (September 1990): 625–30.

22   J. V. Pinkerton, J. H. Pickar, K. A. Ryan, et al., "Conjugated Estrogens and Bazedoxifene in Minority Populations: Pooled Analysis of Four Phase 3 Trials," *Menopause* 23, no. 6 (June 2016): 611–20.

23   S. Palacios et al., "A 7-Year Randomized, Placebo-Controlled Trial Assessing the Long-Term Efficacy and Safety of Bazedoxifene in Postmenopausal Women with Osteoporosis: Effects on Bone Density and Fracture," *Menopause* 22, no. 8 (August 2015): 806–13.

24   "Denosumab," National Cancer Institute, last modified October 23, 2014, cancer.gov/about-cancer/treatment/drugs/denosumab.

Chapter 8: The Estrogen Fix and Your Vagina, Bladder, and Skin

1   M. B. Mac Bride, D. J. Rhodes, and L. T. Shuster, "Vulvovaginal Atrophy," *Mayo Clinic Proceedings* 85, no. 1 (January 2010): 87–94.

2   C. S. Stika, "Atrophic Vaginitis," *Dermatologic Therapy* 23, no. 5 (September–October 2010): 514–22.

3   S. H. Lindahl, "Reviewing the Options for Local Estrogen Treatment of Vaginal Atrophy," *International Journal of Women's Health* 6 (March 13, 2014): 307–12.

4   M. L. Krychman, "Vaginal Estrogens for the Treatment of Dyspareunia," *Journal of Sexual Medicine* 8, no. 3 (March 2011): 666–74.

5   R. E. Nappi and M. Kokot-Kierepa, "Women's Voices in the Menopause: Results from an International Survey on Vaginal Atrophy," *Maturitas* 67, no. 3 (November 2010): 233–38.

6   D. W. Sturdee, N. Panay, and the International Menopause Society Writing Group, "Recommendations for the Management of Postmenopausal Vaginal Atrophy," *Climacteric* 13, no. 6 (December 2010): 509–22.

7   P. Gartoulla et al., "Moderate to Severe Vasomotor and Sexual Symptoms Remain Problematic for Women Aged 60–65," *Menopause* 22, no. 7 (July 2015): 694–701.

8   N. E. Avis et al., "Longitudinal Changes in Sexual Functioning as Women Transition through Menopause: Results from the Study of Women's Health across the Nation," *Menopause* 16, no. 3 (May–June 2009): 442–52.

9   M. Krause et al., "Local Effects of Vaginally Administered Estrogen Therapy: A Review," *Journal of Pelvic Medicine and Surgery* 15, no. 3 (May 2009): 105–14.

10 L. Cardozo et al., "Meta-Analysis of Estrogen Therapy in the Management of Urogenital Atrophy in Postmenopausal Women: Second Report of the Hormones and Urogenital Therapy Committee," *Obstetrics and Gynecology* 92, no. 4 (October 1998): 722–27.

11 "The Role of Local Vaginal Estrogen for Treatment of Vaginal Atrophy in Postmenopausal Women: 2007 Position Statement of the North American Menopause Society," *Menopause* 14, no. 3 (2007): 357–69.

12 N. J. Alexander et al., "Why Consider Vaginal Drug Administration?" *Fertility and Sterility* 82, no. 1 (July 2004): 1–12.

13 Ibid.

14 D. De Ziegler et al., "The First Uterine Pass Effect," *Annals of the New York Academy of Sciences* 828 (September 26, 1997): 291–99.

15 The American College of Obstetricians and Gynecologists, "Committee Opinion Number 659: The Use of Vaginal Estrogen in Women with a History of Estrogen-Dependent Breast Cancer," March 2016.

16 Estring (estradiol vaginal ring) [package insert], New York, NY: Pharmacia and Upjohn Company, division of Pfizer Inc.

17 Vagifem (estradiol vaginal tablets) [package insert], Princeton, NJ: Novo Nordisk Inc.

18 Femring (estradiol acetate vaginal ring) [package insert], Rockaway, NJ: Warner Chilcott (US), LLC.

19 D. Robinson and L. Cardozo, "Estrogens and the Lower Urinary Tract," *Neurourology and Urodynamics* 30, no. 5 (June 2011): 754–57.

20 "What I Need to Know about Bladder Control for Women," National Institute of Diabetes and Digestive and Kidney Diseases, last modified June 29, 2012, niddk.nih.gov/health-information/health-topics/urologic-disease /urinary-incontinence-women/Pages/ez.aspx.

21 O. Contreras Ortiz, "Stress Urinary Incontinence in the Gynecological Practice," *International Journal of Gynaecology and Obstetrics* 86, supplement 1 (July 2004): S6–16.

22 T. Hillard, "The Postmenopausal Bladder," *Menopause International* 16, no. 2 (June 2010): 74–80.

23 C. S. Iosif et al., "Estrogen Receptors in the Human Female Lower Urinary Tract," *American Journal of Obstetrics & Gynecology* 141, no. 7 (December 1, 1981): 817–20.

24 Hillard, "The Postmenopausal Bladder," 74–80.

25 J. A. Fantl, L. Cardozo, and D. K. McClish, "Estrogen Therapy in the Management of Urinary Incontinence in Postmenopausal Women: A Meta-Analysis. First Report of the Hormones and Urogenital Therapy Committee," *Obstetrics and Gynecology* 83, no. 1 (January 1994): 12–18.

26 P. Luthje et al., "Estrogen Supports Urothelial Defense Mechanisms," *Science Translational Medicine* 5, no. 190 (June 19, 2013): 190 ra 80.

27 B. Eriksen, "A Randomized, Open, Parallel-Group Study on the Preventive Effect of an Estradiol-Releasing Vaginal Ring (Estring) on Recurrent Urinary Tract Infections in Postmenopausal Women," *American Journal of Obstetrics & Gynecology* 180, no. 5 (May 1999): 1072–79.

28 C. Y. Long et al., "A Randomized Comparative Study of the Effects of Oral and Topical Estrogen Therapy on the Lower Urinary Tract of Hysterectomized Postmenopausal Women," *Fertility and Sterility* 85, no. 1 (January 2006): 155–60.

29 I. Goldstein and J. L. Alexander, "Practical Aspects in the Management of Vaginal Atrophy and Sexual Dysfunction in Perimenopausal and Postmenopausal Women," *Journal of Sexual Medicine* 2, supplement 3 (September 2005): 154–65.

30 Ibid.

31 P. M. Sarrel, "Effects of Hormone Replacement Therapy on Sexual Psychophysiology and Behavior in Postmenopause," *Journal of Women's Health & Gender-Based Medicine* 9, supplement 1 (2000): S25–32.

32 S. L. Hendrix et al., "Effects of Estrogen with and without Progestin on Urinary Incontinence," *JAMA* 293, no. 8 (February 23, 2005): 935–48.

33 J. Fantl et al., "Estrogen Therapy in the Management of Urinary Incontinence in Postmenopausal Women: A Meta-Analysis. First Report of the Hormones

and Urogenital Therapy Committee," *Obstetrics & Gynecology* 83, no. 1 (January 1994): 12–18.

34 American Society for Aesthetic Plastic Surgery, "The American Society for Aesthetic Plastic Surgery Reports Americans Spent Largest Amount on Cosmetic Surgery Since The Great Recession of 2008," (March 20, 2014): surgery.org/media/news-releases/the-american-society-for-aesthetic-plastic-surgery-reports-americans-spent-largest-amount-on-cosmetic-surger.

35 G. S. Ashcroft and J. J. Ashworth, "Potential Role of Estrogens in Wound Healing," *American Journal of Clinical Dermatology* 4, no. 11 (2003): 737–43.

36 T. Inoue et al., "The Role of Estrogen-Metabolizing Enzymes and Estrogen Receptors in Human Epidermis," *Molecular and Cellular Endocrinology* 344, no. 1–2 (September 15, 2011): 35–40.

37 M. J. Thornton, "The Biological Actions of Estrogens on Skin," *Experimental Dermatology* 11, no. 6 (December 2002): 487–502.

38 R. Maheux et al., "A Randomized, Double-Blind, Placebo-Controlled Study on the Effect of Conjugated Estrogens on Skin Thickness," *American Journal of Obstetrics & Gynecology* 170, no. 2 (February 1994): 642–49.

39 E. D. Son et al., "Topical Application of 17Beta-Estradiol Increases Extracellular Matrix Protein Synthesis by Stimulating TGF-Beta Signaling in Aged Human Skin In Vivo," *Journal of Investigative Dermatology* 124, no. 6 (June 2005): 1149–61.

40 E. F. Wolff, D. Narayan, and H. S. Taylor, "Long-Term Effects of Hormone Therapy on Skin Rigidity and Wrinkles," *Fertility and Sterility* 84, no. 2 (August 2005): 285–88.

41 M. Brincat et al., "Skin Collagen Changes in Postmenopausal Women Receiving Different Regimens of Estrogen Therapy," *Obstetrics and Gynecology* 70, no. 1 (July 1987): 123–27.

42 M. Brincat et al., "Long-Term Effects of the Menopause and Sex Hormones on Skin Thickness," *British Journal of Obstetrics and Gynaecology* 92, no. 3 (1985): 256–59.

43 Brincat et al., "Skin Collagen Changes," 123–27.

44 Ibid.

45 P. Affinito et al., "Effects of Postmenopausal Hypoestrogenism on Skin Collagen," *Maturitas* 33, no. 3 (1999): 239–47.

46 R. Maheux et al., "A Randomized, Double-Blind, Placebo-Controlled Study on the Effect of Conjugated Estrogens on Skin Thickness," *American Journal of Obstetrics & Gynecology* 170, no. 2 (February 1994): 642–49.

47 A. V. Sauerbronn et al., "The Effects of Systemic Hormonal Replacement Therapy on the Skin of Postmenopausal Women," *International Journal of Gynaecology and Obstetrics* 68, no. 1 (January 2000): 35–41.

48 Brincat et al., "Skin Collagen Changes," 123–27.

49 J. B. Schmidt et al., "Treatment of Skin Aging with Topical Estrogens," *International Journal of Dermatology* 35, no. 9 (September 1996): 669–74.

Chapter 9: The Estrogen Fix for a Fit, Energized Body

1   "Obesity and Overweight," World Health Organization, last modified January 2015, who.int/mediacentre/factsheets/fs311/en.

2   P. Pajunen et al., "Metabolically Healthy and Unhealthy Obesity Phenotypes in the General Population: The FIN-D2D Survey," *BMC Public Health* 11 (2011): 754.

3   Ibid.

4   C. C. Wee, R. B. Davis, and M. B. Hamel, "Comparing the SF-12 and SF-36 Health Status Questionnaires in Patients with and without Obesity," *Health and Quality of Life Outcomes* 6 (2008): 11.

5   M. Bogenrief, "Retailers Can't Ignore 100 Million Plus-Size American Women Forever," *Business Insider*, December 21, 2012, businessinsider.com/why-isnt-plus-size-bigger-2012-12.

6   B. Sternfeld et al., "Physical Activity and Changes in Weight and Waist Circumference in Midlife Women: Findings from the Study of Women's Health across the Nation," *American Journal of Epidemiology* 160, no. 9 (November 1, 2004): 912–22.

7   J. R. Guthrie, L. Dennerstein, and E. C. Dudley, "Weight Gain and the Menopause: A 5-Year Prospective Study," *Climacteric* 2, no. 3 (1999): 205–11.

8   S. R. Davis et al., "Understanding Weight Gain at Menopause," *Climacteric* 15, no. 5 (2012): 419–29.

9   Ibid.

10 Ibid.

11 K. Sutton-Tyrrell et al., "Reproductive Hormones and Obesity: 9 Years of Observation from the Study of Women's Health across the Nation," *American Journal of Epidemiology* 171, no. 11 (June 1, 2010): 1203–13.

12 C. H. Kroenke et al., "Effects of a Dietary Intervention and Weight Change on Vasomotor Symptoms in the Women's Health Initiative," *Menopause* 19, no. 9 (September 2012): 980–88.

13 N. H. Rogers et al., "Reduced Energy Expenditure and Increased Inflammation Are Early Events in the Development of Ovariectomy-Induced Obesity," *Endocrinology* 150, no. 5 (May 2009): 2161–68.

14 M. E. Jones et al., "Aromatase-Deficient (ArKO) Mice Accumulate Excess Adipose Tissue," *Journal of Steroid Biochemistry and Molecular Biology* 79, no. 1–5 (December 2001): 3–9.

15 R. E. Stubbins et al., "Oestrogen Alters Adipocyte Biology and Protects Female Mice from Adipocyte Inflammation and Insulin Resistance," *Diabetes, Obesity and Metabolism* 14, no. 1 (January 2012): 58–66.

16 K. M. Flegal et al., "Prevalence and Trends in Obesity among US Adults, 1999–2008," *JAMA* 303, no. 3 (January 20, 2010): 235–41.

17   M. J. Toth et al., "Menopause-Related Changes in Body Fat Distribution," *Annals of the New York Academy of Sciences* 904, (May 2000): 502–6.

18   S. Santosa and M. D. Jensen, "Adipocyte Fatty Acid Storage Factors Enhance Subcutaneous Fat Storage in Postmenopausal Women," *Diabetes* 62, no. 3 (March 2013): 775–82.

19   K. L. Shea et al., "Body Composition and Bone Mineral Density after Ovarian Hormone Suppression with or without Estradiol Treatment," *Menopause* 22, no. 10 (2015): 1045–52.

20   B. L. Wajchenberg, "Subcutaneous and Visceral Adipose Tissue: Their Relation to the Metabolic Syndrome," *Endocrine Reviews* 21, no. 6 (December 2000): 697–738.

21   I. Janssen et al., "Menopause and the Metabolic Syndrome: The Study of Women's Health across the Nation," *Archives of Internal Medicine* 168, no. 14 (July 28, 2008): 1568–75.

22   J. Abdulnour et al., "The Effect of the Menopausal Transition on Body Composition and Cardiometabolic Risk Factors: A Montreal-Ottawa New Emerging Team Group Study," *Menopause* 19, no. 7 (July 2012): 760–67.

23   S. C. Ho et al., "Menopausal Transition and Changes of Body Composition: A Prospective Study in Chinese Perimenopausal Women," *International Journal of Obesity* 34, no. 8 (August 2010): 1265–74.

24   D. H. Morris et al., "Body Mass Index, Exercise, and Other Lifestyle Factors in Relation to Age at Natural Menopause: Analyses from the Breakthrough Generations Study," *American Journal of Epidemiology* 175, no. 10 (May 2012): 998–1005.

25   R. J. Norman, I. Flight, and M. C. Rees, "Oestrogen and Progesterone Hormone Replacement Therapy for Peri-Menopausal and Post-menopausal Women: Weight and Body Fat Distribution," *Cochrane Database of Systematic Reviews,* no. 2 (2000): CD001018.

26   H. Yuksel et al., "Effects of Oral Continuous 17Beta-Estradiol Plus Norethisterone Acetate Replacement Therapy on Abdominal Subcutaneous Fat, Serum Leptin Levels and Body Composition," *Gynecological Endocrinology* 22, no. 7 (July 2006): 381–87.

27   C. K. Sites et al., "The Effect of Hormone Replacement Therapy on Body Composition, Body Fat Distribution, and Insulin Sensitivity in Menopausal Women: A Randomized, Double-Blind, Placebo-Controlled Trial," *Journal of Clinical Endocrinology and Metabolism* 90, no. 5 (May 2005): 2701–7.

28   Z. Chen et al., "Postmenopausal Hormone Therapy and Body Composition—A Substudy of the Estrogen Plus Progestin Trial of the Women's Health Initiative," *American Journal of Clinical Nutrition* 82, no. 3 (September 2005): 651–56.

29   S. R. Davis, K. Z. Walker, and B. J. Strauss, "Effects of Estradiol with and without Testosterone on Body Composition and Relationships with Lipids in Postmenopausal Women," *Menopause* 7, no. 6 (November–December 2000): 395–401.

30   Chen et al., "Postmenopausal Hormone Therapy," 651–56.

31   C. M. dos Reis et al., "Body Composition, Visceral Fat Distribution and Fat Oxidation in Postmenopausal Women Using Oral or Transdermal Oestrogen," *Maturitas* 46, no. 1 (September 25, 2003): 59–68.

32   A. J. O'Sullivan et al., "The Route of Estrogen Replacement Therapy Confers Divergent Effects on Substrate Oxidation and Body Composition in Postmenopausal Women," *Journal of Clinical Investigation* 102, no. 5 (September 1, 1998): 1035–40.

33   E. Sonnet et al., "Effects of the Route of Oestrogen Administration on IGF-1 And IGFBP-3 in Healthy Postmenopausal Women: Results from a Randomized Placebo-Controlled Study," *Clinical Endocrinology* 66, no. 5 (2007): 626–31.

34   D. E. Bonds et al., "The Effect of Conjugated Equine Oestrogen on Diabetes Incidence: The Women's Health Initiative Randomised Trial," *Diabetologia* 49, no. 3 (March 2006): 459–68.

35   S. K. Phillips et al., "Muscle Weakness in Women Occurs at an Earlier Age Than in Men, but Strength Is Preserved by Hormone Replacement Therapy," *Clinical Science* 84, no. 1 (January 1993): 95–98.

36   M. Brown, "Skeletal Muscle and Bone: Effect of Sex Steroids and Aging," *Advances in Physiology Education* 32, no. 2 (June 2008): 120–26.

37   R. C. Griggs, "Effect of Testosterone on Muscle Mass and Muscle Protein Synthesis," *Journal of Applied Physiology* 66, no. 1 (January 1989): 498–503.

38   S. Sipila et al., "Effects of Hormone Replacement Therapy and High-Impact Physical Exercise on Skeletal Muscle in Post-Menopausal Women: A Randomized Placebo-Controlled Study," *Clinical Science* 101, no. 2 (2001): 147–57.

39   S. M. Greising et al., "Hormone Therapy and Skeletal Muscle Strength: A Meta-Analysis," *Journals of Gerontology, Series A: Biological Sciences and Medical Sciences* 64A, no. 10 (October 2009): 1071–81.

40   D. R. Taaffe et al., "The Effect of Hormone Replacement Therapy and/or Exercise on Skeletal Muscle Attenuation in Postmenopausal Women: A Yearlong Intervention," *Clinical Physiology and Functional Imaging* 25, no. 5 (September 2005): 297–304.

41   G. F. Maddalozzo et al., "The Effects of Hormone Replacement Therapy and Resistance Training on Spine Bone Mineral Density in Early Postmenopausal Women," *Bone* 40, no. 5 (May 2007): 1244–51.

42   L. R. Simkin-Silverman et al., "Lifestyle Intervention Can Prevent Weight Gain during Menopause: Results from a 5-Year Randomized Clinical Trial," *Annals of Behavioral Medicine* 26, no. 3 (December 2003): 212–20.

43   commonfund.nih.gov/hmp/index.

44   L. Yurkovetskiy et al., "Gender Bias in Autoimmunity Is Influenced by Microbiota," *Immunity* 39, no. 2 (August 22, 2013): 400–12.

45   B. J. Fuhrman et al., "Associations of the Fecal Microbiome with Urinary Estrogens and Estrogen Metabolites in Postmenopausal Women," *Journal of Clinical Endocrinology & Metabolism* 99, no. 12 (December 2014): 4632–40.

46   G. Williams, "Gut Bugs' Relationship with Estrogen-Related Cancer," The Mix at UAB, November 29, 2012, themixuab.blogspot.com/2012/11/gut-bugs -relationship-with-estrogen.html.

47   C. S. Plottel and M. J. Blaser, "Microbiome and Malignancy," *Cell Host & Microbe* 10, no. 4 (October 20, 2011): 324–35.

48   K. Ravella et al., "Chronic Estrogen Deficiency Causes Gastroparesis by Altering Neuronal Nitric Oxide Synthase Function," *Digestive Diseases and Sciences* 58, no. 6 (June 2013): 1507–15.

49   A. Pan et al., "Bidirectional Association between Depression and Type 2 Diabetes Mellitus in Women," *Archives of Internal Medicine* 170, no. 21 (2010): 1884–91.

50   R. A. Wild et al., "CHD Events in the WHI Hormone Trials: Effect Modification by Metabolic Syndrome. A Nested Case/Control Study within the WHI RCTs," *Menopause* 20, no. 3 (March 2013): 254–60.

51   K. L. Margolis et al., "Effect of Oestrogen plus Progestin on the Incidence of Diabetes in Postmenopausal Women: Results from the Women's Health Initiative Hormone Trial," *Diabetologia* 47, no. 7 (July 2004): 1175–87.

52   Ibid.

53   R. I. Pereira, B. A. Casey, T. A. Swibas et al. "Timing of Estradiol Treatment after Menopause May Determine Benefit or Harm to Insulin Action," *Journal of Clinical Endocrinology & Metabolism* (October 1, 2015).

Chapter 10: Talking to Your Health-Care Provider about Estrogen and the Estrogen Fix

1   R. P. C. Kessels, "Patients' Memory for Medical Information," *Journal of the Royal Society of Medicine* 96, no. 5 (May 2003): 219–22.

2   Ibid.

3   J. L. Anderson et al., "Patient Information Recall in a Rheumatology Clinic," *Rheumatology* 18, no. 1 (February 1979): 18–22.

4   T. P. Canavan and N. R. Doshi, "Endometrial Cancer" *American Family Physician* 59, no. 11 (June 1, 1999): 3069–76.

5   G. Opolskiene, P. Sladkevicius, and L. Valentin, "Prediction of Endometrial Malignancy in Women with Postmenopausal Bleeding and Sonographic Endometrial Thickness ≥ 4.5 mm," *Ultrasound in Obstetrics & Gynecology* 37, no. 2 (February 2011): 232–40.

6   H. Devlin et al., "The Role of the Dental Surgeon in Detecting Osteoporosis: The OSTEODENT Study," *British Dental Journal* 204, no. 10 (May 24, 2008): E16.

7   cancer.gov/about-cancer/causes-prevention/risk/diet/vitamin-d-fact-sheet.

Index

Underscored page references indicate sidebars and tables. **Boldface** references indicate illustrations.

A

Abbreviations guide, 4, 5
Abdominal exercises, 183–84
Abdominal fat. *See* Belly fat; Visceral fat
Actonel, for osteoporosis treatment, 152
Acupuncture, 66
Adhesive patches, 46, 47–48, 48
Alcohol
    bone loss from, 150–51
    breast cancer risk from, 37–38, 73, 80
Alternative menopause therapies, 35, 59–61
    complementary medicine, 66–69
    herbal and plant-based, 61–65
    for mental health issues, 117
    prescription medications, 69–71
    tips about, 60–61
    vaginal moisturizers, 66
    vitamins, 65–66
Alzheimer's disease
    contributors to, 79, 102, 103, 105, 106, 110–11, 124
    estrogen and, 37, 39, 104, 121–24
AMH test, indicating perimenopause, 22
Androgen hormones
    converted to estrone, 27–28
    in women vs. men, 29
Androstenedione, menopause and, 29, 30
Antibiotics, 165, 180
Antidepressants
    for depression, 112–13, 116, 117
    for increasing serotonin, 118
    lower libido from, 117
    for menopausal symptoms, 31, 69–70, 70
Anti-Müllerian hormone level, indicating perimenopause, 22
APOE-e4 gene, Alzheimer's risk and, 124

Aromatization, estrogen produced by, 27–28, 106
Arterial plaque, 87–88, 95, 96, 97, 103
Aspirin, for reducing heart disease, 99
Associate activation, for sleep improvement, 134
Atrophic vaginitis, 70, 154, 155

B

Bacteria
    intestinal, 118–19, 179, 180, 181, 183, 185
    in probiotics, 165
    UTIs from, 163, 165
    vaginal, 154, 179
Balance exercises, 185
Bazedoxifene. *See* Duavee
Belly fat
    diabetes and, 181
    estrogen and, 174–75, 176, 179
    menopausal, 171, 173, 176, 179
    reducing, 183–84, 185
Binosto, 152
Bioidentical hormones
    estrogen, 27–28, 47
    overview of, 51–54
    progesterone, 44, 57
    TX-001HR, 44
Bioidentical pellets, 49–50
Birth control, during perimenopause, 32
Bisphosphonates, for osteoporosis, 143, 151–52
Black box warnings, on estrogen, 36, 53, 74, 158
Black cohosh, 60, 61, 62
Bladder. *See also* Incontinence
    estrogen window for, 153, 161, 164, 170
    sensitive, 159–60, 165

Irritability, menopausal, 107, <u>114</u>, <u>115–16</u>, 119, 127
IUD, progesterone-secreting, 57, 79

J

Jolie, Angelina, 78–79

K

Kronos Early Estrogen Prevention Study (KEEPS), 98–100

L

Lactobacillus
  for UTI prevention, 165
  in vagina, 154, 179
LDL cholesterol, 46, 87, 88–89, **88**, 90
Leptin, 127
Libido loss
  causes of, 1, 30, 61, 83, <u>117</u>
  estrogen preventing, 100
Life span, increased, 9–10, <u>33</u>, 83
Lipid profile, 89
Lipids, 87
Liver, processing oral estrogen, 46, 90, 177, 180

M

Magnesium
  for bone growth, 137
  for osteoporosis prevention, <u>142</u>, <u>151</u>
Major depressive disorder, 119, 120
Maki, Pauline, interview with, <u>113–17</u>
Mammograms, 58, 76, 77, <u>81</u>, 192
Mayer-Rokitansky-Küster-Hauser syndrome, 157
McIndoe procedure, 157
Medroxyprogesterone acetate (MPA). *See* Provera
Memory, 104, 105, 106
Menarche, 18
Menopausal hormone therapy (MHT), <u>5</u>
Menopausal symptoms. *See also specific symptoms*
  antidepressants for, 31, 69–70, <u>70</u>
  duration of, 30–31
  effect on workplace, 128–33, 136
  estrogen for, 2, 14

impact of, 14
lifestyle changes and, 71
non-estrogen therapies for, 61–71
types of, 1, 5, 154–57
Menopause
  average age of, 40
  breast changes in, 76–77
  definition of, 19, 23
  depression in, 35, 39, 111–13, <u>114–15</u>, <u>116</u>, <u>117</u>
  early or premature, 29–30, 34–35, 39–40, 79, 103, 109–10, 141
  estrogen reduction in, 1–2, 22, 28, 31
  facts about, 23, <u>23</u>
  heart disease and, 94–96
  induced or iatrogenic, 23
  mood changes during, 5, 69, 107–11, <u>113–17</u>, 119–20, <u>121</u>, <u>123</u>
  natural or spontaneous, 23
  reflections on, <u>24–26</u>
  sarcopenia after, 177
  surgical, <u>6</u>, 23, 29, 34–35, 79, 94–95, 105, 109, 139
  testosterone reduction in, 29, 30
MenopauseBreakthrough.com, 133, 163
MenopauseQuiz.com, <u>22</u>, 71, 161, 195
Menstrual cycle, 18, 75
Metabolic syndrome, 175, <u>175</u>, 181, <u>185</u>
"Metabolic Syndrome Song," 175
MHT, <u>5</u>
Microbiome, gut, 179–81, 183, <u>186</u>
Microvascular heart disease, <u>92</u>, 93–94
Mirena IUD, 57
Mood changes
  in menopause, 5, 69, 107–11, <u>113–17</u>, 119–20, <u>121</u>, <u>123</u>
  in perimenopause, 21, 22
MPA. *See* Provera
Muscle loss, from aging, 177–79, <u>184</u>

N

Natural hormone therapy, definition of, 51
News avoidance, at bedtime, <u>134</u>
Night sweats
  lifestyle changes reducing, 31
  in menopause, 5, 31, 44, 125, 127, <u>127</u>
  patient story about, <u>31</u>
  treatments for, 50, 60, 61, 63, 64, 66, 113, <u>117</u>

Norethisterone acetate, 56, 96
Nurses' Health Study, 95, 96, 182

O

Obesity
  health risks from, 27, 28, 38, 171
  sarcopenic, 177–79
Oblique muscles, strengthening, 183–84
Omega-3s, for skin care, 166–67
Oral estrogen therapy
  belly fat and, 176–77
  for better sleep, 134
  blood clots and, 38, 46, 47, 55, 57, 90
  blood glucose and, 90, 177
  cholesterol and, 46, 88, 90
  dosages of, 37, 40, 45, 46
  heart disease and, 177
  for osteoporosis prevention, 148, 149
  processed by liver, 46, 90, 177, 180
  skin thickness and, 169
  tablets, 45–46
  types of, 36, 37
  vaginal estrogen vs., 157–58, 163, 164
Ospemifene, 70
Osphena, 70
Osteoblast cells, in bone building, 138
Osteoclast cells, in bone breakdown,
  138, 147, 152
Osteopenia, 138, 139, 141, 145
Osteoporosis
  Brisdelle and, 70
  causes of, 138, 139
  facts about, 140–41
  fractures from, 37, 138, 140, 141, 145
  medications for, 149–52
  preventing, with
    calcium, 113, 142–43, 144–46, 151
    Duavee, 57
    estrogen, 147, 148–49, 149
    lifestyle changes, 142–43, 150–51
    nutrients, 113, 142, 144–47, 151
  risk factors for, 35, 39, 141
  testing for (see Bone density test)
  tooth loss with, 193
  vaginal ring and, 50
Ovarian cancer, 78, 79, 81, 81, 191
  hysterectomy preventing, 29, 30, 110
Ovaries, hormone production in, 2, 27,
  28, 29
Overweight, health risks from, 171

P

Painful intercourse
  estradiol levels and, 164
  incidence of, 40
  Osphena for, 70
  prasterone for, 71, 160
  from vaginal atrophy, 154, 155–56,
    156
Pancreatic cancer, 79, 81, 193
Pap test, 191, 192
Parkinsonism, 104
Parkinson's disease, 79, 104, 109
Paroxetine, 69
Patches. See Adhesive patches
Patient stories
  brain health, 108–9, 108, 111
  heart attack, 92
  hot flashes and chest pain, 91
  hot flashes and night sweats, 31
  mood swings, 121, 123
  osteopenia, 145
  painful intercourse, 156
  skin appearance, 168
  sleep problems, 126, 127
  symptoms from surgical menopause,
    6
  UTIs, 162
Paxil, 69, 70
Pellets, estrogen, 49–50, 52
Pelvic exam, 190–92
Pelvic ultrasound, 44, 57, 191, 192
PEPI (Postmenopausal Estrogen/
    Progestin Interventions) Trial,
    11
Perimenopause
  depression in, 112, 113
  emotional changes in, 107, 119
  estrogen use in, 2, 36
  facts about, 18–19, 21–23
  hormonal fluctuations in, 2, 2, 22, 28
  pregnancy during, 31–32
  reflections on, 24–26
  seeking help for, 31
  sleep problems in, 125, 126
  symptoms of, 19, 19, 21
  testing for, 22
Planks (exercise), 184
Plaque, arterial, 87–88, 95, 96, 97, 103
PMS, 109, 115, 116, 119, 121
Positivity, for sleep improvement, 134–35

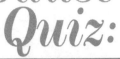
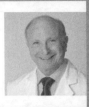
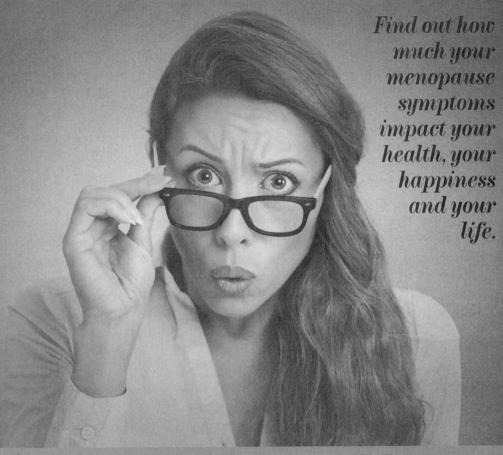